Dr. Romano's

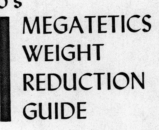

MEGATETICS
WEIGHT
REDUCTION
GUIDE

Dr. Romano's

MEGATETICS WEIGHT REDUCTION GUIDE

Ronald R. Romano, D.C.

Parker Publishing Co., Inc.
West Nyack, N.Y.

Library of Congress Cataloging in Publication Data

Romano, Ronald R
   Dr. Romano's Megatetics weight reduction guide.

   Includes index.
   1. Reducing--Psychological aspects. 2. Reducing
exercises. 3. Reducing diets. I. Title.
II. Title: Megatetics weight reduction guide.
RM222.2.R63 1977   613.2'5   77-12420
ISBN 0-13-217091-4

Dedication

To Joan, your patience is appreciated

A WORD FROM THE AUTHOR

As you begin to read the following pages, you will quickly find that the Megatetic Weight Reduction Guide is a revolutionary new approach to the problem of obesity. Never before has it been possible to lose so many pounds, so quickly, and so easily.

As you proceed through the various chapters you will learn how Megatetics controls the three basic causes of overweight. Not just one or two, but all three causes are taken into consideration and treated, so as to produce amazing results in an extremely short time. You will also find that the Megatetic Weight Reduction Guide is more than just a book to be read and put aside; but rather, a complete program . . . a weight reduction kit, to be utilized, and referred to often as you go about melting away those unwanted pounds.

From the very first moment that you begin your weight reduction program, you will find the daily schedules to be of enormous value as they relate, step by step, what you are experiencing and how you should be feeling. You will be amazed at the rapidity with which you lose weight; overjoyed when you find yourself reaping the benefits of exercise without exercising. And once you learn about the safe, inexpensive tablet that not only helps you lose weight but also maintain your lower weight, you'll be truly excited; especially since this tablet can be purchased at any pharmacy without a prescription.

But all this is only a part of the Megatetic Weight Reduction Guide. Since Megatetics is a complete program, you will also be shown how to enjoy yourself while staying slender. And you'll love the Energy Expender, which forces you to use up those extra calories without even thinking about it. You'll learn how others who were overweight have used the Megatetic Program successfully. But best of all you'll learn how to accept yourself as the new slender

7

person you are, and begin to enjoy every day as an active, interesting individual that others like to be around.

Because of this, I would like to ask you to disregard any prior conceptions you may have about dieting. If you will but follow the directions as outlined, you will be amazed at the results obtained . . . and all this will occur in 30 days or less.

I therefore wish you happiness and good health on this, the first day of your new slender life.

Ronald R. Romano, D.C.

CONTENTS

1 | HOW THE MEGATETIC PROGRAM DIFFERS FROM OTHER DIETS

If you are like most of the overweight patients I've treated, you are probably asking yourself how Megatetics differs from other dietary programs. In this chapter I hope to present information which will demonstrate the reason Megatetics is unique, and why it has been so successful.

Before reading on, though, you should understand that the principles incorporated in the Megatetic Weight Reduction Guide are based on accepted scientific findings. The results of physiological, biochemical and kinesiological studies have been combined in the Megatetic program in a manner intended to produce dramatic weight loss in a very short time.

The case of Barbara R. is a perfect example of how Megatetics works. When Barbara first sought out help for her weight problem, she was 28 years old and weighed 187 pounds. She had been overweight as long back as she could remember, and had tried many different diets and exercises. Barbara had strikingly beautiful features ... but her overlarge body detracted enormously from her looks.

I put Barbara on the 30 day rapid weight-loss program and gave her some specific pointers about energy expenders (a unique method of burning up calories without exercise). In just one month Barbara lost 43 pounds.

To say the least, she was enthusiastic. During the program she had so much energy that she painted and redecorated her apartment all by herself. In addition, she went out and bought a sewing machine so she could design and make her own clothing. When next I saw Barbara, she was radiant. Her new figure and enhancing clothes, combined with her natural attractiveness, produced a remarkably beautiful young woman.

Results such as these are commonplace. Thirty pounds in as many days is the rule, not the exception. When the need exists to lose even 50 pounds in one short month, Megatetics has proven successful ... time and time again. If you wish to join the numerous patients who have found a new, slender way of life through Megatetics, read on.

Since some of the statements contained in the following pages will seem unusual, or perhaps complex, be sure to re-read those portions which you don't completely understand. This will result not only in immediate success regarding weight loss, but also in long-term maintenance of your lowered weight.

THE ORIGIN OF MEGATETICS

During my years as Director of Clinical Services at the Cedars Health Center it has been my responsibility to consult with, examine, and diagnose each new patient. In addition, I have been responsible for formulating therapeutic (treatment) programs for these patients based on the findings of my examinations. In most cases the results of these therapy programs have been excellent, but in some cases patients fail to respond to therapy. It was through my concern for these "failures" that I discovered a method by which patient control could be increased. This method is based on positive feedback mechanisms and a detailed explanation of the various components of any particular therapy program.

When this method was used, the results of therapy increased proportionately. Numerous patients with complex disorders began to show improvement. The benefits of therapy became apparent and I was more than satisfied with the results. Shortly after implementation of this new method, however, I discovered that many overweight patients continued to fail to lose weight on what was then considered to be an excellent dietary program. This was incongruous! Why were we realizing increased results from patients with varied pathologies, but almost no change in results from weight-reduction patients? I re-examined folders; re-evaluated the dietary program; and spoke to each patient who had failed to lose weight. After numerous consultations I began to notice similarities among the various comments and criticisms about the diet then in use. There seemed to be three major complaints:

1) The weight loss wasn't large enough,
2) The diet took too long, and
3) The exercises were boring.

In addition to these complaints almost every patient reported that they "knew" that even though they continued on the diet to completion they would never be able to live the rest of their lives eating only the foods listed in the program, especially in the amounts specified.

I took these complaints seriously. I began to formulate a weight-loss program that overcame the stated objections. During the months that I was preparing a new dietary program—I continued to examine and diagnose new admissions. One afternoon, after having completed my examination of an intelligent, middle-aged businessman, I found myself discussing with him, his thoughts about success.

He maintained that success was nothing more than a demonstration of the truth contained in the phrase—"Survival of the fittest." He felt that only those individuals who were "fit" in a business sense could survive the rigors necessary for success. For some unknown reason this statement remained in my mind. As I continued to work on my dietary program, I found myself correlating survival with obesity. A few days passed and at one point I discovered myself picturing overweight and underweight individuals competing for survival in a prehistoric environment. Under these imaginary conditions it seemed self-evident that the underweight person would soon succumb to the rigors of life and the lack of food, while at the same time the individual who was overweight in today's society would probably reduce his weight and adapt to the environment sufficiently.

This, then, was my first realization that in today's society the fittest (healthiest) individuals are overweight. It became apparent that due to the lack of strenuous physical exertion and the overabundance of food, healthy individuals would conserve maximum amounts of energy in the form of fat, while those individuals with relatively inefficient digestive systems would barely maintain proper weight levels even though they consumed large quantities of food.

It seemed ironic that a society which had been built by the fit and strong was now acting to the detriment of those very same individuals. Yet this was exactly what had happened, and this was what had to be taken into consideration if obese individuals were to reduce their weights and prolong their lives. The Megatetic Weight Reduction Program was founded on this primary concept.

THE TRUE CAUSE OF OBESITY

During the time that you have been overweight, I am sure you have heard people say that obesity is unhealthy. It is common knowledge that a fat person's life expectancy is much shorter than if he were of "normal" weight. These statements are true and their implications are serious.

Numerous individuals, including some physicians, believe that obesity is a disease. Others say that overweight individuals are gluttonous; that they overeat, and that this is the reason they are fat. Still others believe that you, and all fat people, are lazy; that you refuse to perform physical tasks and therfore do not utilize the calories which you consume. These statements are false, and no matter how many times they are repeated, or how adamantly they are defended, they will remain false.

The true cause of your overweight condition is HEALTH*, not sickness. By this I mean that although obesity is in itself unhealthy, the cause of obesity is not.

HOW HEALTHY PEOPLE BECOME OVERWEIGHT

Health is considered to be physiological. That is to say that health is nothing more than the proper and efficient functioning of all the various organs and systems of the body.

Since we are not presently concerned with medical disorders unrelated to obesity, let's focus our attention on the physiological activity of the gastrointestinal (digestive) tract as it relates to your overweight condition. Consider for a moment that you were to eat a small piece of candy that contained 100 calories. If, through the proper functioning of your digestive tract, you absorbed and utilized or stored most of these calories you would be said to be healthy at least with regard to your digestive system. If, on the other hand you did not absorb a major portion of the calories, but rather allowed many of them to pass through your body unused, you would be considered "sick". Your digestive system would not be functioning properly because it was incapable of utilizing the full complement of calories which you had ingested. From this simple example it can be seen that the healthy individual would absorb more calories from the food he eats than would the "unhealthy" individual.

The above example does not, of course, reflect on all the various physiological processes of your body. It is certainly true that overweight individuals can suffer with disorders unrelated to the cause of obesity.

HOW CALORIC ABSORPTION CONTROLS OBESITY

Calories are nothing more than units of energy contained in the food we eat. These units of energy are absorbed through the digestive process, and if there is an oversupply of them in our

---

*At this point I am not referring to the rare case of glandular pathology which results in extreme obesity. The vast majority of overweight individuals are considered to be physiologically healthy relative to the cause of their overweight condition. It is to these individuals that I address myself.

bloodstream our bodies will store them in the form of fat for future requirements. Since healthy people absorb more of their food's calories and nutrients, it can easily be seen that they will have increased numbers of energy units in their bloodstreams. Over the years the healthy person builds up an increasingly large reserve of these units in the form of fat, and this eventually leads to obesity. It is in this way that the healthy person becomes overweight.

By the same token, the individual whose physiological processes are not performing properly, will not absorb as many calories from his food and therefore will not have sufficient reserves in the bloodstream. Thus there will be little or no storage in the form of fat.

HOW YOUR EFFICIENCY CAN LEAD
TO A SLENDER BODY

In the previous paragraph I explained how healthy people become overweight through increased absorption of food. This, however, is not the only cause of your overweight condition. When we speak of health as it relates to obesity, we must consider all its various aspects. Digestion and absorption of food is only one of the numerous physiological processes which are constantly in operation in your body. If we can objectively consider your body as a work machine, you will easily understand that the more efficiently it operates, the healthier it is. The rapid and complete absorption of food is a good example of this efficiency as it relates to internal chemical processes. It is also true, however, that any outward physical activity you perform can also be measured in degrees of efficiency. Therefore, if we were to consider two individuals accomplishing the same tasks, we would be able to rate them according to how efficiently they perform. For example, let's consider two men who have been assigned the task of digging a hole two feet wide and two feet deep. The first man positions himself properly. He holds his shovel in both hands, minimizes the amount of flexion in his spine, uses the weight of his body to penetrate the upper layers of compacted earth, and places the excavated dirt nearby. He works smoothly and rhythmically to accomplish this task. The second man crouches over his work; he uses the strength in his arms and back to break through the dirt. He changes his posture continuously and discards the excavated material so close to his work that he will have to move it again in order to produce the correct diameter hole. From this example it is easy to see which man works more efficiently and uses less energy to achieve the same end. The first man not only conserves energy, but also accomplishes his task more rapidly. He is therefore considered to be the more efficient of the two.

It is apparent therefore, that there must be some innate mechanism which affects the way certain individuals approach physical work. If you will spend some time observing how others accomplish various tasks, you will note that slender individuals use up excessive energy and make numerous wasted motions when performing even the simplest activity. At the same time, overweight individuals generally seem to accomplish several tasks with increased efficiency, and therefore with a much lessened expenditure of energy.

The point I am making here is that overweight is the result of both increased absorption in the digestive tract and the efficient operation of the musculo-skeletal system. It therefore becomes apparent that certain healthy individuals obtain increased calories from their food, while at the same time using up fewer calories through physical activity. This produces an overabundance of calories in the bloodstream with resultant storage deposition in the form of fat.

HOW MYLA H. LOST 37 POUNDS

Myla H. had been a patient of the Center for several years. Except for occasional problems that required treatment, she came in only once a year for a complete examination. Each time I examined Myla I remarked about her overweight condition, but apparently she was not interested in losing weight as she never responded to my advice in this area. One day as I was performing an annual physical on Myla she broke down and began to sob. As I questioned her to determine what was wrong, Myla responded, "It's unfair! Why do I have to be overweight? My husband eats just as much as I do and he never gains a pound. My sister, too! She eats everything; sweets, cake, bread—and yet she's as thin as a rail. It's unfair that I have to be fat."

Once I had calmed her down, I explained that the reason she was overweight was because she was healthy. She stared at me in amazement and I could see that she didn't understand what I meant.

"You see, Myla," I continued, "you have probably been taught to believe that something is wrong with you, that you suffer from some as yet undiscovered disease or deficiency. Perhaps you even believe that you somehow are at fault for your obesity. This couldn't be further from the truth.

"Let's compare you and your husband just for a moment. The fact is, that although your husband eats as much as you, he never gains weight. This is due to an inability to properly absorb the nutrients contained in the food he eats. Much of what he eats passes right through his digestive system and he gains no benefit from it. On the other hand your body is working properly. It absorbs as much as possible of the nutrients from the food you eat, and since you aren't as active as you used to be, those extra calories you're absorbing are showing up on your body in the form of fat instead of being burned off.

"But Dr. Romano, what am I going to do?" Myla asked. "I try to cut down on my food but it doesn't seem to help. I lose a couple of pounds and then I gain them right back."

I explained the Megatetic Program to Myla, being sure that she understood every part of it. The following week, after her examination results had been analyzed, she began on her 30-day program. For the first time in her life Myla was enthusiastic about losing weight. She no longer felt that she had been born to be fat. Myla completed the program on schedule. In only 30 days Myla lost 37 pounds, and through continued use of the Megatetic Principle she maintains this substantial weight loss even today, three years after completing her program.

A DIFFERENCE THAT RESULTS IN GREATER WEIGHT LOSS

Every dietary program I have ever seen disregards the fact that overweight people absorb more of the nutrients and calories from their food than do their more slender counterparts. Instead, the major emphasis is placed on the quantity or quality of the food consumed. In almost every diet, portions must be measured, calories counted or food lists consulted, to determine whether or not a particular food can be eaten. This wouldn't be half so horrible if the diet was fast and effective. In most cases though, the overweight individual loses only small amounts of weight. Months and sometimes even years are required to achieve a desirable weight level. This is truly unfortunate because most overweight people can achieve a desirable weight in one month or less. There is no need to spend vast amounts of time analyzing menus or preparing special foods. And once you have achieved your desirable weight you should be able to maintain it without the necessity of leading a monastic life.

Other dietary programs I've seen also include exercises in their regimen in an effort to use up the excess calories that overweight people absorb. It has been my finding however, that overweight individuals detest exercises which are performed just for the purpose of losing weight.

It is the rare individual indeed who relishes the thought of rolling around on the floor, attempting gymnastic feats that were meant for circus performers. Twisting, gyrating, bending and pulling, all in a last ditch effort to reduce the size of a waist or thigh. It is my belief that the only exercises that are of value are the ones which can be continued for life without the need of special equipment or prescribed times for their performance. Too many of the exercise programs I've seen are restrictive, time consuming, and generally worthless when considered in the light of rapid and dramatic weight reduction.

The Megatetic Weight Reduction Guide, on the other hand, is different in that it is designed to produce the largest amount of weight loss in the shortest possible time. Not only is the quantity and quality of the food you eat taken into consideration but also increased energy expenditure is built into the program without the use of routine, strenuous exercises. In addition, the Megatetic program incorporates a method by which absorption in the digestive tract is reduced. Therefore, the number of calories you get from your food is also reduced, and this results in fewer calories being available in your bloodstream. Since each of these factors is equally important, and since the Megatetic Weight Reduction Program takes them all into consideration, the result is the fastest and easiest weight-reduction program available.

THE MEANING OF MEGATETICS

The Megatetic Dietary Program has produced excellent results. The combination of methods which produces large weight losses in extremely short time is better than any other program I've encountered. It would seem that for some reason the results which are produced through this program exceed what could normally be expected. More weight is lost than on any diet, and it is lost more quickly than on any exercise program. In fact, it would appear that the various portions of this dietary program come together to produce a synergistic effect. Thus the benefits of each portion of the program are increased because of its interaction with every other portion. It is for this reason that the term Megatetics is used to describe this approach to rapid weight loss. Mega—which comes from the Greek word *megas*, means great or mighty and—tetics is from the word dietetics which is the science of applying the principles of nutrition. In this way, the term Megatetics conveys the fact that this program is greater in its results than either dietetics or exercises alone.

THE NOT-UNUSUAL STORY OF PAM L.

I am presenting the following case history not only because it is typical of so many patients I have seen, but also because I feel that Pam's experience will help you realize the true benefits of weight reduction. The problems that Pam faced are probably very similar to your own. I truly hope that by relating her story I will stimulate you to make up your mind to lose weight.

When Pam first consulted me she was complaining of chronic neck pain and continuous dull headaches. Not once did she refer to her obesity although she was 31 pounds overweight. At 29 years of age she looked old and sad. Her hair, which was cut short, made her round face appear much heavier than it actually was. Her skin was

THE MEGATETIC PRINCIPLE

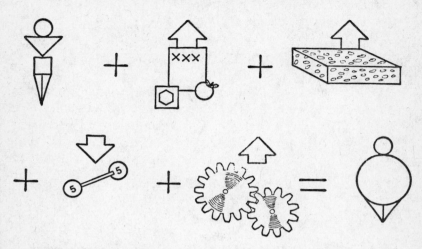

FIGURE 1-1: *Depicts a normal individual who eats more food than is required for health. In addition, he absorbs more of the nutrients contained in the food while at the same time he performs less physical activity. These facts, plus increased efficiency, lead to obesity.*

pale and she wore no makeup. Her clothing was little different from the kind I had come to expect on overweight patients—dark drab colors, one or more sizes too small for her overlarge body.

During our first consultation, I noted that Pam was forcing herself to be cheerful. She responded to my questions in an off-handed way—trying to make light of her neck discomfort as well as any other subject which came up. She responded quickly, almost defensively to questions about herself. By the end of our first interview I had discovered that Pam was divorced, and had been so for the past four years; that she worked at an exclusive restaurant in the Palm Beaches as a bookkeeper; and that she had no children and lived alone. Her medical history was inconclusive as were her physical, laboratory and X-ray examinations. It was therefore concluded that her neck and headache problem was probably due to postural

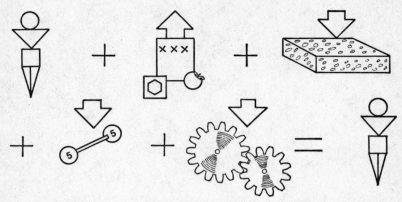

FIGURE 1-2: Depicts a normal individual who also eats more *food than necessary but does* not *absorb as much of the nutrients contained in the food. Even though this individual performs little physical activity, he does so with decreased efficiency and therefore maintains a "normal" weight.*

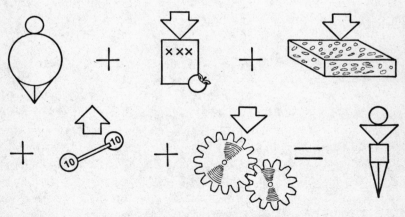

FIGURE 1-3: Depicts an overweight individual who, by decreasing food intake and absorption, increasing the amount of physical work performed, and at the same time reducing his efficiency, produces a rapid loss of weight.

disorders relative to her work. I made a few simple suggestions regarding proper posture and re-scheduled her for a follow-up office visit in two weeks. The time of her appointment came and passed, but Pam didn't return.

Several weeks later Pam once again called for an appointment. When she came in she told me that she had followed my instructions and that she was no longer bothered by neck pain or headaches. Since she had felt OK she didn't bother to keep her follow-up appointment. Pam appeared to be in better spirits than on her first visit. She reported that she had been quite impressed with her rapid improvement and that since I had made the suggestion that she lose some weight she was going to "give me a try."

This second consultation was much more revealing. Pam told me quite a bit about herself. She told me that while she was married she had become pregnant but lost the baby in her sixth month. She felt that this miscarriage had contributed to her later divorce. For some unknown reason, Pam revealed more about her true feelings on this second office visit than any other patient I can recall. She told me of her loneliness, her feelings of depression, and her infrequent but frightening periods of despair. At the conclusion of our visit, I felt that I had known Pam for a long time, although we had not spent more than an hour together.

Her childhood and teenage years, her unsuccessful marriage, the trauma of miscarriage, her repeated failure to lose weight, had all led Pam to believe she was worthless. Another appointment was made for the following day; a third consultation would be necessary.

When Pam returned, I investigated further into her lifestyle and especially her eating habits. I learned that Pam routinely skipped breakfast except for a couple of cups of coffee. During the remainder of the morning she would consume several more cups of coffee but no solid food. At lunch she would usually have a rather large and over-rich meal. The afternoon would find her consuming several more cups of coffee. Upon returning home in the evening she would have two and sometimes even three alcoholic drinks followed by a variety of "meals"—usually pre-packaged foods of little nutritional value. I was amazed at her apparent good health in spite of her injudicious behavior. Potato chips, cookies, coldcuts, canned fruit, TV dinners, and bread were her NORMAL fare. We spent considerable time on this third interview, but when it was over Pam recognized her true situation. She realized that not only was her obesity a result of earlier events, but also that it was a cause of present emotional and psychological distress. Pam agreed that her overweight condition was a hindrance to her own happiness, and that she would follow my every instruction for the next 30 days.

As I look back at that first day of Pam's program I can still recall my feeling that she was challenging me; that she really didn't believe she could ever lose weight. I must admit however, that Pam lived up to her word and did everything she was supposed to. She followed instructions to the letter and although she often felt sorry for herself she refused to let her feelings interfere with her program.

Pam found the first few days the most difficult, but as she reported to me later, "she had made up her mind to lose weight". Her initial motivation, stimulated by a rapid weight loss (12 pounds the first three days) was more than enough to keep her on the right track. By the sixth day her visual goals had become part of her. She could see how she was going to look in only a few short weeks. As the days continued to pass and Pam's weight continued to drop, she took on a new appearance, a new attitude. She was happy, excited about her future prospects. By the ninth day her previously too tight clothes had become too baggy. She began to write up a list of the clothes she would buy when her 30-day program was over. Her appearance improved considerably and she started to spend a few extra minutes with her hair and makeup. Initially she had been skeptical, but now as the Energy Expenders became more and more a part of her everyday activities, Pam was certain she was on the right road to slenderness. Her personality changed at the same time. Her response to questions was no longer overly quick. She became subdued, quiet and confident in herself. She smiled more and spoke with true feeling; without continuous jokes or cynical remarks. In 24 days she reached her desired weight. She had lost 31 pounds.

From that point on a new life began for Pam. It was as if there had been an age regression...with each pound lost, Pam had become younger. She now went out and bought the wardrobe she had wanted: New, bright colors, form-fitting skirts and blouses, sweaters, slacks—and even new shoes because the ones she had were now too loose on her feet. She began to cater to herself. She made time for the hairdresser, frequently indulged in the luxury of facials, and manicures. She took membership in a local health club, not for the purpose of losing additional weight, but rather for the enjoyment she obtained from the swimming pool, sauna and steambath. Her outlook had changed remarkably during the short period of the program. She realized that she had a basic worth and she became proud of her accomplishment. Even her employer noted the change, and when she requested additional duties he was the first to recognize the benefit of having her greet patrons. Pam no longer spends her days in a small room, hidden from view, working on the books. She is out front, greeting guests, enjoying new and interesting people.

It has been 18 months since Pam took hold of herself and "made up her mind to lose weight". Her life has changed dramatically. She faced her problems and overcame them. And although it was difficult, Pam now has achieved a new and exciting lifestyle. She is happy and content with herself and her surroundings. The loss of only 31 pounds made Pam's life worth living.

2 | HOW MEGATETICS WORKS

M ost overweight individuals spend considerable time trying to lose their excess pounds. Every time a new fad, pill, or injection is announced, they are there, ready to try it—willing to do almost anything to reduce their weight. Unfortunately, after trying several different diets and taking numerous pills or injections, they become discouraged and depressed. There seems to be no way for them to permanently reduce their weight and they therefore give up all hope of ever being slender. Fortunately, all is not lost! The reason you and others like you have not been successful in the past is because you have never had the reasons for your obesity properly explained.

If you are like the majority of overweight individuals, you have probably come to believe that the only reason you are fat is because you overeat. Although excessive intake of food is definitely a part of the obesity syndrome, it is by no means the *only* part. Controlling the quantity of food you eat, although important, will not result in rapid or sustained weight loss. If you are to be successful, you will have to take into consideration *all* of the reasons for your obesity.

THE 3 REASONS YOU ARE OVERWEIGHT

As is the case in most conditions affecting humanity, obesity cannot be considered as the result of only one causative factor. Instead, it should be understood that your overweight condition stems from three primary causes. These are:

1) the quality, as well as the quantity, of the food you eat,
2) the absorption and utilization of the nutrients you consume, and
3) your psychomotor efficiency.

Unless, and until, all these factors are taken into consideration, any attempts to permanently lose weight will eventually meet with failure.

HOW THE QUALITY AND QUANTITY OF FOOD YOU EAT AFFECTS YOUR WEIGHT

Each of the various foods you eat differs in the quality of nutrients it contains. You are most likely aware of the fact that some foods contain more calories than others. This, to some extent, affects the relative quality or value of the food. More importantly, however, there are factors contained in all foods which must be taken into consideration in any dietary program. I am referring here to the specific nutrients found in varying amounts in proteins, carbohydrates and fats. These specific nutrients, the essential amino acids, oils, vitamins and trace elements are more directly related to the quality of a specific food than are calories. If your normal dietary intake does not contain sufficient and properly balanced amounts of these necessary elements, the quality of the foods you eat is poor. Your body is not receiving adequate quantities of the elements necessary to sustain life and rebuild tissue properly. In most cases however, you are probably eating just enough of these essential nutrients to preclude the appearance of any full-blown disease syndrome. This, then, results in what are known as subclinical deficiencies—deficiencies which are not dramatic enough to produce fully recognizable symptoms. In any event, the deficiencies *do* exist. Since you are not consuming the proper quality foods, your body begins to crave additional quantities of the poor quality foods you do eat. In this way you begin to eat larger and larger amounts of food in an effort to correct the underlying deficiencies. Unfortunately though, the food you eat contains little, if any, of the nutrients you are lacking because in all likelihood it is the same food which produced the original, deficient state. It is in this way that the quality of the food you eat leads to increased quantities of food desired, with a resultant increase in calories consumed. These increased calories cannot be properly utilized by your body and are therefore deposited as fat in the intercellular spaces.

HOW GEORGE C. BENEFITTED THROUGH A CHANGE IN DIET

When George C. first consulted me, he was complaining of chronic low back pain. He was 33 years of age and weighed 231 pounds. At the time, he was employed as as a carpenter and therefore expended considerable physical energy while working. I examined George and found that his low back pain was due to an instability of the lumbo-sacral articulation. This is the last freely movable articulation at the base of the vertebral column. On further questioning, George admitted that he was also concerned about bruising easily. He reported that even slight trauma resulted in black and blue marks on almost any part of his body.

Since it was going to take a few days for us to get back the results of our laboratory tests, I asked George to complete a dietary analysis for us in the meantime. George was advised to write down everything he drank or ate for the next few days, so that we could evaluate his food intake. When the laboratory results were returned, nothing of major significance could be found. George was recalled to the office at which time I checked his dietary analysis. From what George had written down, I could see that he was a "meat and bread" man. His intake of fruits, vegetables and dairy products was negligible. Sandwiches, and especially beef, were his mainstay. He was eating huge quantities of meat but little else of nutritional value. By putting together the findings of my examinations with his food intake data, it was easy to see that George was suffering from several vitamin deficiencies. I called this to his attention and pre-scribed therapeutic doses of several nutritional supplements. I felt that the instability of his low back was due to ligament laxity, which caused excessive mobility of the articulation, resulting in pain. Since Vitamin C is always indicated when there is involvement of the connective tissues, I prescribed extra large doses of this factor. George was re-scheduled for one month, at which time I would perform a re-evaluation. When he came in, he reported that his low back discomfort was markedly reduced and also that he noticed he wasn't bruising as easily as before. Apparently, the high doses of Vitamin C, and other supplements had not only increased the strength of the vertebral ligaments but had also strengthened the capillary walls of the vascular system (blood vessels). George was pleased with the results and requested that I help him lose weight. He was placed on the Megatetic Program and lost 47 pounds. To-day, George continues to perform physical labor—but his food in-take is properly balanced. He no longer suffers with back discomfort or bruising, and reports that he feels much more energetic since paying attention to the quality as well as the quantity of the food he eats.

YOUR MIRACULOUS DIGESTIVE TRACT

In order to best understand how your increased ability to absorb nutrients from food results in obesity, let's look at how your diges-tive tract works.

The digestive tract (also known as the alimentary canal) begins at the lips, proceeds through the mouth and esophagus to the stomach, and then finally through the intestines to the anus. It is more than 30 feet in length and has as its primary function the breaking down and absorption of nutrients.

Very little of the food you eat can be directly absorbed into the bloodstream and it is therefore the job of the digestive tract to break the various nutrients down into simpler molecules so that the body can utilize them.

In the previous section I mentioned the factors which are re-

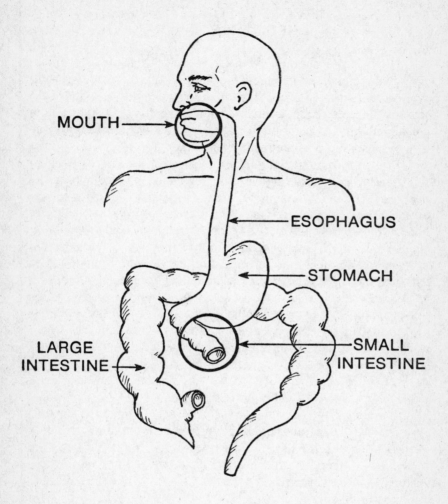

FIGURE 2-1: THE DIGESTIVE TRACT.

sponsible for altering the quality of the food you eat. At this point it is important for you to understand the differences between protein, carbohydrate and fat.

HOW THE VARIOUS FOOD COMPONENTS
AFFECT YOUR HEALTH

No matter what food you eat, it consists of either protein, carbohydrate or fat. Although butter looks and taste different from, say, olive oil, they are basically the same since they are both pure fats. By the same token, almonds and milk are alike in that they both contain all three of the primary materials. Almonds and milk consist of a combination of proteins, carbohydrates and fat.

Protein is found mainly in meat, fish and fowl. It is essential to human life because the amino acids of which it is composed are necessary to rebuild the muscular, neurological and osseous tissues of our bodies. Without protein in our diet, and our body's ability to break it down and absorb the component amino acids, we would soon die. Carbohydrate and fat do not contain the essential amino acids which are necessary to rebuild the protein in our own bodies and therefore they cannot replace protein in our diet.

Carbohydrate is usually found in the form of sugar or starch and comes mainly from vegetable products. You will find carbohydrates in all fruits and vegetables as well as in the products which are made from them (i.e., bread, cakes, etc.).

Fat, on the other hand, is found in both animal products (i.e., cream, butter and egg yolk, as well as the fat on meat) and in vegetables such as olives, cottonseeds or peanuts.

Generally, we can think of fat and carbohydrate as the fuel necessary to keep our bodies going, while protein is primarily needed to rebuild the tissues. In any event, all three materials are necessary for good health and the factors which compose these materials must be absorbed into the bloodstream before we can benefit from them.

If you can imagine trying to push a pearl through a sieve, you will immediately realize the importance of the digestive process. The pearl is much too large and therefore cannot pass through the small openings in the sieve. If, however, we were to first pulverize the pearl with a hammer so that it became a fine powder, we could easily see how it would then pass through without difficulty. In this same way the food we eat is composed of molecules too large to pass through the walls of the digestive tract. The molecules must be split into very small components by means of the digestive process in order to be of value to our bodies. This is accomplished by what are known as enzymes. Enzymes are specific chemicals found within the alimentary canal, capable of splitting large, complex food molecules into small and easily absorbed constituents.

Enzymes are found primarily in the mouth, stomach and small intestines, and it is mainly in these three portions of the digestive tract that food is prepared for absorption into the bloodstream.

The Mouth

The saliva which is secreted into the mouth is composed mainly of water. However, there are small amounts of an enzyme known as ptylin also present. The major function of ptylin is in the initial stages of starch (one form of carbohydrate) digestion. And although this first stage in the digestive process is important, it is overshadowed by the relatively complex digestive processes which occur in the stomach and intestine.

The Stomach

The stomach secretes three important enzymes (i.e., pepsin, rennin, lipase). Pepsin is responsible for the initial breakdown of the protein we eat, but it must first be activated by hydrochloric acid. At the same time, rennin curdles milk, and lipase which is also secreted in the stomach, has the ability to digest fats.

At this point in the alimentary canal, we can see that the protein, carbohydrate, and fat we eat have, at least to some extent, been partially digested. However, the main digestive process occurs in the small intestine. It is in this portion of the digestive tract that the final stages of digestion and absorption occur. All the enzymes necessary for the final utilization of the nutrients we ingest (as well as other chemical components) are found in the small intestines.

Without going into unnecessary detail, you can easily understand that only a healthy individual will be capable of producing sufficient enzymes for complete digestion and absorption. Also, it is equally important for the food to remain in the various portions of the digestive tract for specific periods of time thus allowing total breakdown of the complex molecules into smaller absorbable components. This, too, is relevant when we consider that many slender individuals exhibit increased movement of food through the alimen tary canal. This is definitely not as nature intended and, of course, leads to poor absorption of the nutrients.

It can, therefore, be seen that a normally healthy digestive system is one that secretes sufficient amounts and strengths of the necessary enzymes and retains the food we eat for an adequate time to permit complete digestion and absorption. It is in this way that a healthy individual gains more from his food and therefore becomes overweight.

In order to overcome, at least to some extent, the ability of the overweight individual to more rapidly digest and more completely absorb the nutrients in his food, a simple, yet effective, method had to be devised. It was essential that for the time the method was to be used it be safe and have no major side effects, nor in any way be detrimental. It was only with these thoughts in mind that the Megatetic Tablet, which is easily obtainable in any drugstore, was decided upon.

WHAT BARBARA H. SAYS ABOUT THE MEGATETIC TABLET

Originally, use of the Megatetic Tablet was intended to help decrease the degree of digestion which takes place in the normal, healthy, digestive tract. At the same time, if possible, it was desira ble to alter the amount of time that food would remain in the various parts of the alimentary canal so as to impede absorption and utiliza tion.

When Barbara H. first consulted me about her overweight, I realized that she was a compulsive eater. Not only did she exhibit the results of all the primary causes of obesity but after questioning her, I found that she was a non-stop food machine. She was con tinuously "picking". If it wasn't a cookie, it was a piece of cheese, or a stick of chewing gum. In any case, her mouth was always working on something.

I knew that if we were to help Barbara, we would have to overcome her apparent need to keep eating. We placed her on the standard Megatetic Program, but with little hope of success. It seemed useless! In 30 days Barbara lost 42 pounds and continued to lose during the post-program period. I was amazed—it was as if she had had no problems—apparently something had happened which appeased her need to keep eating. I questioned her about this and she told me that it was all due to the Megatetic Tablet. Not only had it apparently done everything I said it would but also it had somehow satisfied her desire to "chew or eat something". Further investigation revealed that Barbara had used the Tablet faithfully—her timing was exceptional and she had never forgotten to take it. Barbara stated that the initial phase of the program had been difficult for her, but when she saw how quickly the pounds were melting away, she resolved to stick it out. After her 30-day program was so successful, she found herself starting to wonder about the future, but once she began to use the Megatetic Tablet before each meal, she no longer concerned herself about her previous need to eat. Barbara continued to lose weight, and today says that "the Megatetic Tablet turns tubs into Twiggys".

HOW EFFICIENCY CONTROLS WEIGHT

In the previous sections I have presented information which illustrates how the quantity and quality of food as well as your ability to digest and absorb it, produces obesity. Another equally important factor is what is known as psycho-motor efficiency. I touched on this subject in the preceding chapter when I spoke about increasing your energy expenditure, but it is so important that a detailed explanation of it is necessary.

Consider, if you will, the following hypothetical problems. Imagine each step you would take to solve them. Problem F is for the ladies. Problem M for the gents.

Problem F: "I want to make potatoes for dinner this evening. What must I do?"

or

Problem M: "I want to replace the screening in my patio door. What must I do?"

Before looking at the several possible solutions I have given below, try to think out exactly what you would do to solve the problem. Be honest with yourself and then look at the solutions I've given. Try to match your answer as closely as possible to one of the solutions I have given.

Solution

Problem F: If you are like most overweight individuals, you have probably considered the most efficient method which will result in potatoes for dinner. The following solutions are graded according to efficiency:

100%   Have hubby go to the nearby take-out restaurant and purchase an order of mashed potatoes or french fries.

75%   Open a can of pre-cooked potatoes (or instant mashed) and prepare them.

50%   Boil raw potatoes in their jackets or bake them.

25%   Peel, wash, cut and cook the potatoes then mash by hand.

Solution

Problem M:
100%   Have the Mrs. call the home maintenance company and have them repair the door.

75%   Take the door off and put it in the car. The Mrs. can go to the nearest hardware store and have them repair it.

50%   Order the screening by phone and when it's delivered, do the job yourself.

25%   Go to three different stores - compare the cost of screening, then go to the store with the lowest price - buy the screening and return home and repair it yourself.

As you have probably already admitted to yourself, you don' fall into the 25% efficiency category. If you have found a differen solution to the problems presented or have picked one of the solutions given, it's probably better than 50% EFFICIENT. And it's because of this efficiency that you conserve energy and maintain your weight.

The above examples are neither statistically nor scientifically valid but they do give you some insight into how psycho-motor efficiency exhibits itself. On the surface it would appear that if you chose the most efficient method of solving the problem presented, you would be lazy. This is not so, because many individuals who are overweight will go to great extremes using energy in creative activities. If laziness were to blame, this wouldn't happen. It is my belief that the average overweight individual has a very analytical mind which requires constant stimulation. Simple problems for such a mind require simple solutions. To do more than is necessary is foolish and wasteful, yet if a problem presents itself which is challenging, such a mind will spend hour after hour in an effort to produce a satisfactory solution. The solution will undoubtedly require the least amount of physical energy because that is necessary to make the solution equitable to an efficiency-oriented individual.

As can be seen from the above examples, laziness has little, if anything, to do with the way you approach problems or achieve solutions. Unfortunately, however, the fact that you are efficiency oriented does lead to your expending less energy than other individuals do, performing similar tasks. As was said previously, calories are nothing more than units of energy and since you use fewer of these energy units in performing everyday tasks, you will have more units available in the bloodstream for storage.

Thus, we can see that the quantity and quality of food we eat, our body's ability to digest and absorb the nutrients in the food, and our conservation of energy through psychomotor efficiency all lead to obesity.

THE THREE RULES OF MEGATETICS

In formulating a method which would benefit overweight patients, I found that the complex causes of obesity required a straight-forward solution. It therefore became necessary to explain the reasons behind each individual's obesity. As I continued to work with patients, I noted that many soon forgot the importance of controlling each and every factor responsible for their obesity. In an effort to keep the importance of each cause clearly in mind, I formulated the following three rules which I have found to be extremely beneficial. Since you already know why you are overweight, it is unnecessary to have to memorize the causes; but if you are to achieve your goals of a slender and shapely body, you *must* remember these three rules. Memorize them—and also type them on several small pieces of paper so you will continuously have them before you. Place the pieces of paper in strategic locations around your home—the bathroom mirror and the refrigerator door are obvious locations, but don't forget the dashboard of the car, the face of the kitchen clock, your billfold, etc.

By keeping these three rules constantly in mind you will have no trouble in losing those excess pounds.

THE THREE RULES

Eat Less
Absorb a Little
Expend a Lot

During your 30-day program you will eat very little and you will absorb only a small fraction of what you do eat. At the same time, you will increase your energy expenditure.

Truly, you will lose weight and inches faster than you ever dreamed possible.

HOW FRANK R. TESTED THE MEGATETIC PROGRAM

Frank R. was probably one of the most difficult and confusing patients I have ever encountered. Since his retirement from the New York police department, Frank had put on 28 pounds. For a man 57 years old, Frank was still in good shape, but the additional weight he was carrying was definitely putting a strain on his heart. The combination of retirement inactivity and three full meals a day was slowly taking its toll.

Initially, Frank refused to accept the fact that his overweight condition was potentially dangerous. He refused to consider dieting as a viable alternative to obesity. Instead Frank decided he would initiate an exercise program to help him lose the excess pounds. On three separate occasions I cautioned Frank against any strenuous exercises. I explained to him the dangers of putting too much strain on his unconditioned body. If he was determined to try to lose weight by exercise alone, I suggested a moderate exercise format with a gradual increase in the difficulty factor. Frank would have none of it ... he knew his own capacity, and was sure he would not overdo it. As Frank left the office I had visions of him suffering an acute coronary, but nothing I had said seemed to make an impression on him. Three days later, Frank returned.

"Let's get on with it," he said.

"Get on with what?," I asked.

"The exercises," he responded. "You told me not to overdo it, so I want you to give me a list of the proper exercises."

I spent another half hour with Frank that day. I tried to explain that exercises weren't enough. He would have to diet as well. In addition, I explained the necessity of a reasonable post-program procedure.

"That's not for me," Frank responded, as he stomped out of the office again.

I thought for sure I would never again see Frank R., but several days later he was back in the office demanding his dietary program.

Once again I spent considerable time explaining the necessity of following my instructions completely. I also advised Frank to consider several ways he might increase his energy expenditure.

"I'll do exercises," he said. "I like doing exercises, they don't bother me."

"Fine," I agreed. "Here's a list of several rather easy exercises. Follow the instructions and you won't have any problems. If you perform the exercises routinely, and as outlined, they will take the place of your Energy Expender.

"But remember, Frank," I cautioned, "if you don't continue with the exercises you will definitely regain at least a part of the weight you'll soon be losing."

"No problem, Doc," he replied as he left the office.

On his next visit Frank informed me that he had re-arranged all the furniture in his home.

"Why did you do that?" I asked.

"Oh, those exercises you gave me take too much time. I don't want to spend the rest of my life doing exercises," Frank stated.

"Fine, Frank. What other expenders will you be using?" I asked.

"None," he responded, "moving the furniture around will be more than sufficient."

Once again I explained the necessity of following instructions, and once again Frank was certain he knew what had to be done.

During the remainder of the program every suggestion I made was countered by a negative response. Every instruction was either too difficult to comply with or unessential. Each and every time I made a recommendation, it was considered inappropriate. Several times I was on the verge of discharging Frank from my care, but he always managed to come around and follow instructions just in the nick of time.

Frank completed his program successfully and, after following an appropriate post-program procedure for several weeks, was discharged. But that didn't end my consternation regarding Frank's on-again/off-again attitude.

A few weeks ago (more than a year since Frank's last visit to the Center) I got my answer. I was attending one of the local Chamber of Commerces' functions when a woman whom I had never met before came up and introduced herself. She was Frank's wife. After thanking me for taking good care of her husband and helping him to lose weight, she informed me that Frank was still doing quite well with his Energy Expenders and had not regained any of those extra pounds. We talked for a while and during the conversation I remarked on how difficult it had been to convince Frank to do what I knew was best for him.

"Oh that," she replied, "that's normal."

"What do you mean?" I asked.

"Well," she explained, "when Frank was with the (police)

department he worked for Internal Affairs.* He found that during questioning, if he contradicted an officer's statement or disagreed with his point of view, the bad cop would soon alter his statement or at least change the emphasis. A good cop would just ignore the rebuttal and continue with his statement. Frank learned that this technique works equally well outside the department. If he's unsure of himself, not positive what course of action to take in any particular situation, he'll disagree with you and then wait to see if you'll change your statements.

"When he first came to see you he was quite worried about his weight. He'd never before been on a diet and was uncertain as to what would be the best way to handle his weight problem. That's why he kept disagreeing with you and then later following your instructions. He was testing you to see how sure you were of what you were recommending. It's really a crazy way to do things, but Frank's been doing it for so long that I don't think he'll ever change."

---

*A special branch of the police department which is responsible for investigating charges made against police officers.

3 ‖ THE THREE PART PROGRAM FOR SLENDERNESS

30 DAYS TO SLENDERNESS

There are very few dietary programs which can promise substantial weight loss in less than 30 days. Most require several months, or more. It is true that some diets produce marked weight reduction initially— sometimes as much as ten pounds during the first week. Unfortunately though, continuance on these diets rarely produces continued weight reduction. After the first few pounds are lost, a plateau is reached. It makes no difference that the dieter continues to follow instructions and eats only the foods listed. His weight remains steady. After a few more days of sacrifice the average dieter throws up his hands in despair and gorges himself on all the wrong foods— thereby negating any benefit which might have accrued while on the diet.

Once this cycle is repeated several times, the overweight individual becomes failure-oriented. Even though he may start on new diets, he does so with the subconscious knowledge that he will fail. Only a half-hearted attempt is made to lose those extra pounds. Negative thoughts become implanted in the subconscious mind, and even the overweight person begins to believe that slenderness is an unreachable goal.

I must admit that on the surface it does appear unreasonable to expect large numbers of pounds to disappear in only 30 days. It took years to put them on! Day after day and week after week, injudicious diet and lack of energy expenditure gradually increased your weight ounce by ounce. Today, the results of those seemingly unimportant ounces may be evident as extreme obesity. It seems incongruous to expect a rapid reversal, and almost immediate slenderness. Yet, this is exactly what the Megatetic Program is capable of . . . 30, 40, even 50 pounds in less than a month—25 pounds or more the very first week; and the best part about Megatetics is that it can be used for life, thereby permitting permanent slenderness.

If for some reason you are more than 50 pounds overweight—don't worry. Megatetics will produce a 50-pound weight loss each and every month until you achieve your proper weight. If you need to lose less than 50 pounds (but more than 10) you also will find Megatetics faster than any other diet or exercise program you've encountered. If somehow you are only 10 pounds above your desirable weight, then Megatetics will have your weight where it belongs in only seven days (Chapter 8).

Incredible? Yes! But true nonetheless. Not only will all those excess pounds melt away, but so will the inches. During the 30-day program you may have to buy at least one new wardrobe, and probably two. The fat will disappear so quickly that after one week your present clothing will hang on you like so much burlap.

But let's face it—the rapid and enormous reduction in weight and size is only a part of the benefit of Megatetics. More importantly you will be able to maintain your new slenderness for life with only minimal effort. By following the simple procedures listed in the final chapters of this book you will continue to maintain your new found energy levels and the slender body you have desired for so long.

UNDERSTANDING LEADS TO SUCCESS

Every overweight patient I have ever treated has, at one time or another, tried to lose weight by means which can only be described as dangerous. They have attempted to lose weight in much the same manner as they pick their clothing. Whatever was fashionable that season—whatever new fad had hit the magazines—was the way they were going to lose weight. Temporary and partial success was often achieved, but, in the final analysis, failure was inevitable. The reason? Lack of understanding! Either they didn't fully understand what was expected of them or, and this is more commonly the reason, they didn't understand how following a particular regimen would result in weight reduction. Initially, they performed like so many automatons. Their motivation was at a peak. Soon, however, their resolve faltered and they immediately rejected the particular diet, using as a reason their own analysis of its insufficiencies.

As I previously stated, overweight individuals generally have analytical minds. In addition, their intellectual levels are above average. Knowing this, it is easy to understand why fad diets come and go so quickly. They are analyzed out of existence. If every facet of a dietary program is not fully explained or analysis of it does not lead to complete understanding—it will soon be rejected by the analytical mind. It is in this way that lack of understanding leads inevitably to failure. And it is for this reason that I caution you—*do not proceed with the Megatetic Program until you understand each and every part of it*. If, after re-reading and analyzing certain paragraphs, you are still unsure of the rationale—consult your family physician and ask for his assistance—he will be more than happy to oblige. At the same time you should request a complete examination, and should not proceed on *any* diet until you are certain there are no contraindications.

Once you feel confident in your understanding of the Megatetic Program, you will be able to proceed smoothly and rapidly to your final goal . . . a slender body. But don't forget! Megatetics is unique; different from any other diet you've encountered. A complete understanding of why and how it works is essential to your success.

LIMITING FOOD INTAKE FOR RAPID WEIGHT LOSS

Every dietary program, in one way or another, limits food intake. Some diets do this by reducing the quantities of all the various foods you eat. Other diets require that you eat or drink excessive quantities of a particular food or liquid. This, of course, results in a feeling of satiety with a resultant decrease in your consumption of other, and perhaps more desirable, foods, Still other dietary programs restrict your intake of particular kinds of food (i.e., carbohydrates). This, too, results (after initial overindulgence) in a decreased intake of food once your body has consumed sufficient quantities of those foods permitted. On this kind of diet, a point of tolerance is reached after which continued consumption of the permitted foods becomes distasteful if not downright unbearable.

In every case however, every diet, by whatever means, strives to limit your intake of food. Even on those diets which require excessive consumption of a particular item (i.e., grapefruit) the final goal is a decreased consumption of other, more fattening foods.

The major drawback of all these diets is that they become increasingly difficult to follow after the first few days. Initially, when your motivation and resolve are at their highest points, the diet seems fairly easy. After only a short time, however, you begin to crave those foods which are not permitted, or, in the case of those diets which reduce your total intake, you begin to crave larger and larger portions. It is only a matter of time until you fall by the wayside—another dietary failure. Unfortunately, this result—failure, should have been expected. Your response to these types of diets is normal and physiological. The fact that you crave larger portions or portions of those foods which are not permitted, is evidence that your body is working properly. Every time you consume a nutrient, the complex mechanism of digestion and absorption is initiated. Whether you eat one raisin or an entire meal, the chemical, physical and psychological processes of digestion are activated. You begin to crave both physically and psychologically, those foods which have been restricted in your diet. If you had not eaten, you would not have initiated the digestive process and therefore would not have stimulated your appetite. You can therefore see that it would be easier not to eat than to eat small, restricted amounts.

The Megatetic Weight Reduction Program incorporates this basic physiological fact. By controlled abstinence, or fasting, Megatetics produces the rapid weight loss all overweight people want. In addition, however, Megatetics is designed to become easier (not harder) as time goes on. In this way, you will take advantage of your initial motivation while at the same time allowing for a decrease in your resolve during the final days of the program. With only 30 days between you and slenderness, success is assured.

LOSING ADDITIONAL POUNDS BY DECREASING FOOD ABSORPTION

As was said previously, food absorption is just as important as food consumption. If you did not absorb the nutrients you consumed, you would not now be concerned with obesity.

During the first part of your 30-day program food absorption will be insignificant. You will not have to concern yourself with that particular aspect of weight control. At the end of the program, however, and in the future, your ability to absorb the nutrients you consume will have to be altered. This will be done through use of the Megatetic tablet. Your absorption of the various food components will be reduced automatically. You will not have to pay constant attention to your dietary intake because the Megatetic tablet will help you absorb and utilize less. Unlike any other dietary program, Megatetics will assist you when for one reason or another you consume more food than your body requires for normal functioning. Use of the Megatetic tablet will produce results which were previously impossible without the restriction of food intake to a degree that was uncomfortable. You will therefore be able to eat more food than on any other diet, and still continue to lose weight or maintain your proper weight level. You will achieve all this and more by decreasing food absorption through use of the Megatetic tablet

EXPENDING ENERGY WITHOUT EXERCISES

As previously stated, psychomotor efficiency is one of the major causes of your obesity. Through a technique which was developed for my overweight patients, you will begin to burn up more and more calories without routine, standard exercises. As the calories are utilized, pounds will melt away.

By properly programming your daily activities you will automatically expend increasingly greater amounts of energy. This will not only result in greater weight loss but also will increase the tone of your muscles and skin. Therefore, at the end of your program you will have stronger muscles and firmer, more beautiful skin. Your circulatory system will be stronger and your cardiovascular pulmonary reserve (CVP) will have been increased. All in all, your life expectancy will have been lengthened. These benefits, plus the fact that once you have re-programmed your daily activities you will be able to contine to reap these benefits, makes Megatetics the greatest dietary program available. Long after you complete your 30-day program and have attained your desirable weight, Megatetics will continue to work for you in maintaining your slenderness and increasing your life expectancy.

HOW GEORGE T. ADAPTED THE ENERGY EXPENDER TO HIS LIFESTYLE

George T. was 55 years of age and weighed 190 pounds. Because of his short stature he appeared to be much heavier. George was a salesman, and had been one most of his life. His job required him to spend six or seven hours a day just driving, and George believed that it was because of this he was overweight.

After completing the preliminary examinations, George was placed on the Megatetic Program and the Energy Expender was explained to him. His immediate response was that he could not benefit from the Expender. When I asked him why not, he stated that is was impossible to use up extra energy in his kind of work.

Because George appeared to be sincere in his desire to lose weight, I spent considerable time analyzing his daily routine. Apart from those activities common to all of us, George's day appeared to be nothing more than driving to his customers' places of business, going inside, writing up an order, and returning to his car.

Because George had been in business for many years, he knew most of his customers quite well. He did very little selling—most of his work was in writing up re-orders. After discussing this with him, George began to see how he could alter his daily activities.

He took on several extra product lines and put together a sample kit. In addition he began carrying with him small supplies of the most commonly needed products. Each day he made it his business to stop at one new prospective customer, in addition to his usual route. In a short time George's attitude changed. He no longer carried only his order pad when calling on customers. Instead he always brought his sample case with him to demonstrate new products or improvements in old ones. This, of course, resulted in increased business. When customers ran out of a particular item, George gave them an emergency supply from the stock he carried in his car. This, too, resulted in increased business. The extra stops George made each day also paid off. New customers and more orders resulted.

After a few months, George's new routine had become second nature to him. He had taken on a new vitality and interest in his job and his business was excellent. In addition, George had continued to lose weight and achieved his goal the first month. The enormous number of calories which George burned up on a routine basis by changing his daily programming led to rapid and sustained weight loss.

Seeking out new customers, demonstrating his products, carrying a larger line, and the resulting extra business, meant burning up hundreds of calories each day. All without exercises.

4 | HOW LIMITING FOOD INTAKE RESULTS IN RAPID WEIGHT LOSS

The Megatetic Weight Reduction Program is
unique. Not only because of the quick
and sustained weight losses which result from it, but also because it
incorporates all of the proven methods which have been shown to
make weight loss easier.

In this chapter, I will present the single most important dietary
approach essential to permanent weight control. As you proceed
through the Megatetic Program to completion, however, you will be
required to choose certain alternate dietary approaches based on
your particular life style. These will be presented in later chapters
and unless you have a complete and thorough understanding, you
will be unable to choose that approach which is best for you.

Since the first 30 days are completely programmed, it will not
be necessary to concern yourself about them. At the end of the
30-day program you will have lost 40, 50 or more pounds. If additional weight must be lost to achieve your desirable weight level,
you need only follow the directions outlined in Chapter 7.

Once you have achieved your ultimate goal however, it will be necessary for you to maintain it.

The several alternate approaches which will be presented will permit you to do this with little or no effort on your part.

FREEDOM THROUGH FASTING

Centuries before the birth of Hippocrates (the Father of Medicine) fasting was used extensively for the relief and cure of many disorders. Numerous conditions were treated successfully through the judicious use of fasting and it therefore became the primary therapeutic approach of that time.

It was only in recent years that fasting was discarded as a beneficial aid to health. Many physicians, unaware of the results obtainable through fasting, ignored it and relegated it to the ranks of untried therapies.

Today, however, scientific interest in the physiology of fasting is increasing and it is quickly returning to popularity as a therapy of choice, both here and in Europe.

WHY FASTING IS SIMPLE

A true fast is nothing more than a total and complete abstinence from food. You have probably heard of some individual who has been on a juice "fast" (meaning only fruit or vegetable juices were permitted). This of course is inconsistent with the above definition of fasting. Fruit and vegetable juices contain nutrients and are therefore food. One cannot consume food and be said to be fasting at the same time. The only true fast consists of taking nothing but water for varying periods of time, and only a true fast will produce the beneficial and remarkable results you desire. Not only will the pounds rapidly melt away, but you will also realize a new vitality and excitement about life.

HOW FASTING BENEFITS YOUR ENTIRE BODY

Fasting does not really commence until at least 24 hours after your last food consumption. Many individuals who miss a meal or two consider themselves as having fasted. This, however, is untrue. The healthy body requires approximately one full day to completely process any food you eat. Unless and until all nutrients have passed completely through your body, a fasting state has not been achieved. Once this does occur however, the body's physiological processes begin to change. The digestive process, with all its attendant physical and chemical activities, gradually comes to a halt. Since there is nothing to digest, the hydrochloric acid of the stomach, as well as the digestive enzymes of the small intestine, slowly diminish. Elimination is reduced since only non-nutritive residue and bacteria remain in the alimentary canal. A cleansing process begins. Toxins which are present in the bloodstream from over-absorption and under-utilization as well as the remnants of cellular destruction are quickly disposed of. The liver, which during normal times is under constant pressure to cleanse the blood is given partial respite. There is no longer any food being processed through the digestive tract and therefore one of the liver's major duties is temporarily dispensed with. There is now time for the liver to "catch up". The blood circulating through the body contains the debris of old tissue cells and the toxic by-products of chemical reactions necessary for life. In a relatively short time however, the level of toxins in the circulating blood is reduced even though old tissue cells continue to be destroyed. Since nutrients are no longer reaching the liver from the digestive tract, the body turns to its huge reserves of fat for its necessary energy supply. Millions upon millions of fat molecules are broken down and released from the tissue spaces for use by the various organs. Thousands of calories which normally would have been supplied by the food you eat are now supplied from your own fatty tissues as the body begins its purification process. The toxins which are released by fat breakdown are quickly excreted. Since the digestive process has come to a standstill—little, if any, of the various chemicals necessary for digestion have to be replaced. Therefore, other essential chemical components (i.e., hormones and antibodies) which may have been in a depleted state are now manufactured. Tissue cells are replaced at an increased rate, and healing may proceed in rapid fashion. The entire organism benefits as the constant pressure of having to digest, absorb, utilize and store the products of digestion is eliminated. This process continues until such time as you ingest even the smallest amount of food. When this occurs, the processes of fasting are immediately reversed. Digestion, with all its various physical and chemical reactions, is initiated, and the physiological processes integrally associated with it begin again. During the time of the fast, however, much has been accomplished. The reduced weight and the increased vitality remain with you as reminders of the benefit of fasting.

THE ANSWERS TO YOUR QUESTIONS ABOUT FASTING

Many people who have tried to fast on their own have failed miserably. Yet, when properly instructed in what to do and what to expect, they have proceeded without difficulty and achieved their goals in short order.

To preclude any difficulty while you are on your Megatetic program, the following explanations are offered. I have tried to answer patients most commonly asked questions.

> *Every time I miss a meal I get a severe headache. How will I be able to continue on a fast?*

Headaches, which in this case are due to a lowering of the blood sugar levels, can be distressing. They are a normal consequence of restricting food intake. Fortunately, they rarely last for more than a few hours and are self-limiting once your body adapts to a normal blood sugar level. Usually the headache is less severe if the previous meal was not loaded with carbohydrates. Therefore, when beginning on your 30-day program you are cautioned not to overindulge prior to the start of the fast.

In any event, if the headache is not alleviated by resting in a supine position, one or two aspirins with one ounce of milk will usually suffice to make you comfortable until your blood sugar level returns to normal.

> *When I first started on the program, I had a headache but it disappeared overnight. Now I am into my second (or third) day of the program and am being bothered by a constant, dull headache. Why is this?*

Your initial headache was due to blood sugar level deviations. Your present headache, however, is due to toxemia. Your body is presently breaking down reserve fat cells for energy. The toxins released by this chemical reaction are at relatively high levels in your bloodstream and are irritating to the nerve fibers of the vascular system. This causes dilation or enlargement of the blood vessels with resultant headache. As your body adapts to receiving energy from your own fat cells, it will become increasingly proficient in destroying and excreting these toxins, thereby reducing the levels circulating in the blood. As this happens, your headache will gradually disappear. Depending on how toxic you were prior to beginning on your fast, this cleaning may take from one to three days.

After the second day on the program I noticed I had a horrible mouth (and body) odor. I also discovered that my tongue was coated and discolored. What is this from?

As soon as your body was given the chance, it began cleansing itself. The toxic by-products which had built up over many years in your bloodstream and tissues had to be disposed of. The body accomplishes this in several ways. A substantial amount of toxic material is expelled as gases through the pulmonary (lung) fields. At the same time numerous glands which are embedded in the skin also excrete toxic, odoriferous material. This is the cause of the mouth and body odor. You will notice their gradual disappearance as the body fluids are cleansed.

The coating on your tongue is also a sign that the body is ridding itself of undesirable chemicals. Remember as a child how your doctor always checked your tongue when you were sick? By doing this he was verifying the fact that your body was working properly to cleanse itself of whatever was irritating it.

As you continue with your program, your tongue will gradually clear; indicating that your body has been sufficiently cleansed. This is an excellent indication of your progress.

How come I feel so tired and weak?

Tiredness is not uncommon in the initial stages of fasting. It is usually just another side-effect of toxic buildup in the bloodstream. It will soon disappear and be replaced by a feeling of euphoria.

Energy levels will increase to such an extent that you will be completely amazed at what you can physically accomplish. Every patient who has followed the program correctly reports that after initial fatigue and weakness disappear, they have energy to burn and become involved in projects which they had been putting off.

I am always hungry. How can I possibly go without food for a prolonged period of time?

First, you must understand the difference between appetite and hunger. If you crave food several hours after having eaten, you must recognize this as appetite. This is a learned mechanism. It is activated by the clock and not by a true need for food. If you see or smell (or sometimes just visualize) food several hours after eating, your mouth may begin to water. This is a learned response not unlike the response of Pavlov's dog. By refusing to give in to this artificial desire for food—you will soon overcome it. After just one or two days on the program your appetite will be suppressed, and food will hold little, if any, interest for you.

Hunger, on the other hand, is a natural and necessary desire for food. It will not appear until your body has cleansed itself sufficiently and used up most of its reserves. Sometimes hunger doesn't occur at any point during the program because of the manner in which it has been set up. Bear with, and refuse to give in to, your initial craving for food (knowing it is only false appetite) and it will soon disappear.

I have been on the program for several days and I am still having bowel movements. Why is this?

A large portion of any bowel movement consists of bacteria which normally live in the intestinal tract. In addition, the cells which line the alimentary canal are normally sloughed off and also appear in the bowel movement. Since you are no longer eating any food, the size of your bowel movements has decreased. However, the cellular and bacterial components are still being excreted from time to time. This is what makes up the bulk of your movements at the present time.

When I broke the fast according to instructions, I had a watery bowel movement. Is something wrong?

No! It is normal to have a watery stool after being on a fast. It will take the body a few days to readjust to the intake of food. Follow the program as directed and you will not overly irritate the digestive tract.

While on the fast I am being bothered by acid indigestion. What should I do?

Because you are not taking in any food, your body will, from time to time, respond to some sight or mention of food by secreting hydrochloric acid into the stomach. This is normal and can be quickly alleviated by drinking the prescribed fluids. If it should return increase your fluid intake during the day. This will completely neutralize the effects of the acid.

I have never been on a fast, but I have been on many diets. Why do you say fasting is easier?

Not too many years ago there was a potato chip manufacturer who repeatedly used the slogan "Try to eat just one." The psychology behind such a statement is excellent and I am sure resulted in greatly increased sales. By the same token, every diet you have ever been on says "try to eat just this," or "try to eat just this much." The psychological foundations are the same, because it is always more difficult to restrict or limit yourself than it is to abstain completely. This fact can also be demonstrated by, of all things, the standard method of questioning suspects about a crime. Consider for a moment that interrogators first ask the suspect questions which he can easily and truthfully answer without jeopardizing his status. Once he begins to talk about unimportant and nonessential events, it is only a matter of time before he expands into dangerous areas, reporting events which incriminate him.

In the same way, diets which attempt to limit or restrict food intake are rarely successful. If you are permitted to eat and drink, to sit at the dining table, or frequent restaurants, it is only a matter of time before you, too, expand into dangerous areas—eating more than you should or eating foods which negate the effect of the diet.

Fasting, on the other hand, states "I won't have any." Neither that first potato chip nor that first innocuous conversation. I will abstain completely—I will not try to limit myself or attempt to control my appetite—rather, I will deny it completely and abstain totally.

Another factor which makes fasting easier than dieting is physical. Once you begin to eat, you stimulate the physical processes of digestion and the desire for food is increased until the neurological mechanism of satiety is activated by the filling of the stomach. Since fasting precludes the possibility of initiating the digestive process, there is no desire for food, and therefore you can proceed with impunity. Diets lock you into a restrictive and self-immolating lifestyle—only fasting will ever set you free. Free to lose faster than you ever dreamed possible, free to be ... slender and active.

But, Doctor, I can't stay on a fast for the rest of my life—what am I going to do after my 30-day program?

Have no fear! Megatetics is a complete, life-long program. The first 30 days will allow you to achieve your slenderness goals. Each and every day is programmed for you. After you have achieved your desirable weight, the alternate dietary approaches will keep you slender for life. First, you will lose those excess pounds. Then you will stay slender forever. That is why Megatetics is so successful.

Doctor, why is it so important to break the fast in the way that is outlined?

Very simply stated, the improper breaking of a fast not only irritates and possible damages the tissues lining the alimentary canal, but also reverses the beneficial and positive psychological control which you have exhibited while fasting. An oversupply of food, or the taking of improper nutrients can often produce undesirable side effects such as intestinal cramping. Therefore, be sure to follow the recommendations as outlined in the program when breaking your fast.

HOW LOUISE G. FINALLY SUCCEEDED

Louise G. was a middle-aged housewife. Her three children were grown and she was now finding herself unhappy with her obesity. She had been on numerous diets. She had tried shots and pills, but nothing seemed to have any permanent effect. She lost, then gained. Finally, she sought help at the health center.

During her initial 30-day program Louise lost 37 pounds. Since she was extremely overweight a second program was indicated. During her second month she lost an additional 35 pounds—a total weight loss of 72 pounds in just two months.

Today, more than nine months since her program, Louise still maintains her lowered weight. When she recently visited the office, I asked Louise what she thought was the reason for her final success.

"The speed with which I lost weight! I never would have believed I could lose so fast. Over the years, I've tried to diet many times, but always gave up after a short period. I just couldn't accept having to be on a perpetual diet. With the Megatetic Program I knew exactly how long it would take me to achieve my goals. Each day brought me another step closer to where I wanted to be.

"Previously, when I tried dieting I found myself cheating after only a couple of days. It wasn't much; an extra piece of meat or a little bit more vegetable. Unfortunately, though, the cheating became gradually worse until I found myself not losing an ounce.

"I was still paying attention to most of the diet and therefore felt cheated. If I wasn't going to lose any weight, I rationalized, why should I continue to restrict the foods I enjoyed? It was only a matter of a day or two before I disregarded the diet altogether and was back to eating as usual.

"If I had to pick the one thing that helped me be successful, I would say it was this: The speed with which the pounds came off."

5 | MELT FAT AWAY BY REDUCING FOOD ABSORPTION

LIMITING FOOD INTAKE IS NOT
THE COMPLETE ANSWER

As I mentioned previously, every diet you have ever been on tries to limit your food intake in one way or another. The Megatetic Program accomplishes this by the straightforward use of fasting or complete abstinence. There is no great mystery as to the rationale for this approach to dieting. By restricting food intake, fewer calories are available for energy requirements and/or storage. This results in utilization of the body's own fat reserves when energy requirements exceed food intake. In this way the body's fat is rapidly burned up and weight is reduced. In order for most other diets to work, your energy expenditure must remain higher than your food intake. If and when this condition no longer exists you will no longer continue to lose weight. You will reach a plateau and unless you further reduce your caloric intake or increase your energy expenditure, you will have for all intents and purposes, reached the end of your dietary program. Further weight loss is impossible.

The Megatetic Program is designed to prevent stabilization of your weight until you reach your desirable weight goal. By the use of controlled fasting, your energy expenditure can never be less than your food intake. In this way you proceed rapidly and continuously to your lowered weight level and slender body.

Unfortunately, you will not be able to maintain a perpetual fast. Once you have completed your 30-day program you will be returning to those foods you enjoy eating.

In order to maintain your lowered weight while returning to your normal diet, something must be done to prevent over-absorption of the food you eat.

CONTROLLING ABSORPTION CONTROLS WEIGHT

Let us suppose that you have just completed your 30-day Megatetic program. In addition, you have reached your goals on schedule and are presently at your desirable weight. As you return to your usual eating habits, you will have a tendency to overeat. Also, your digestive system, which has had substantial rest during the past 30 days, is ready and capable of absorbing almost any nutrient you ingest. If this is permitted to happen, much of what you have accomplished will be lost. Something must be done to preclude the possibility of your regaining those excess pounds.

One way of accomplishing this is to voluntarily attempt to restrict your food intake. This, however, is difficult, and is the reason most diet programs fail. A voluntary limitation of your food intake is therefore unacceptable.

The only other way to preclude your regaining weight is to reduce absorption and utilization of the food you eat. Since this involves a physiological process and is not under voluntary control, something has to be done to reduce the absorbability of the nutrients which you will be consuming.

In order to accomplish this the Megatetic Tablet will be used for a short period of time. This tablet will reduce the complete absorption of food you eat and therefore will automatically reduce your caloric utilization.

HOW THE MEGATETIC TABLET WORKS
TO PREVENT FOOD ABSORPTION

In a previous chapter I presented material on the physiology of digestion. At that time, I explained that digestion consisted of both a physical and chemical component. The physical portion has to do with the consolidation and movement of food (known as a bolus) through the alimentary canal. The chemical portion is primarily concerned with enzyme activity and the breaking down of food into its component parts so that it is more easily absorbed.

In order to achieve the greatest reduction in the absorption of food, both the physical and chemical components of digestion must be considered and controlled. The Megatetic tablet, which is available at any pharmacy without prescription, accomplishes this. By reducing gastric (stomach) acidity, partially inactivating pepsin (one of the proteolytic enzymes), and producing more rapid emptying of gastric contents, the Megatetic tablet effectively reduces the body's ability to absorb and utilize the food you consume.

As soon as food is introduced into the stomach, the body responds by secreting hydrochloric acid. This is a strong acid capable not only of dissolving organic matter but also certain metals such as iron and zinc. When in proper concentration, the hydrochloric acid of the stomach begins to digest food almost immediately. However, if for some reason there isn't sufficient free hydrochloric acid present, the digestive process will be inhibited. The Megatetic tablet accomplishes this by reducing the acidity (increasing the pH) of the gastric juice through the process known as neutralization. In this way food entering the stomach remains at least partially undigested and therefore unabsorbable.

At the same time that hydrochloric acid is being secreted into the stomach, another chemical, pepsinogen, is also being brought into play. Pepsinogen is a precursor of the enzyme pepsin, and pepsin is primarily responsible for the initial stages of protein digestion. In order for pepsinogen to work, however, it must be activated by hycrochloric acid. Since the Megatetic tablet is capable of neutralizing the hydrochloric acid in the stomach, much of the pepsinogen which is secreted remains in its inactive state. This, of course, results in a further diminishment of digestion with resulting reduction in absorption.

Another, and equally important factor in digestion, is the physical movement of food (bolus) through the digestive tract. In order for the body to complete the digestive process, food must remain in various portions of the tract for specific periods of time. The Megatetic tablet, by neutralizing the gastric contents, causes the stomach to empty sooner than usual. In doing this, the body has less time to act on the food, and therefore cannot completely absorb the nutrients and calories which it contains.

THE MEGATETIC TABLET: WHAT IS IT?

From what has been said previously you are probably thinking that the Megatetic tablet is a new miracle drug only recently formulated. This, however, is not the case. The Megatetic tablet has been available for many years and can be bought at any pharmacy, without a prescription. To my knowledge however, this tablet has never before been used as an aid to weight reduction and it is because of this that I use the term *Megatetic* tablet.

You have probably used these tablets in the past to relieve what is commonly called "indigestion" or "heartburn." The last time you had an upset stomach you probably took one of these Megatetic tablets to alleviate the symptoms. Yet, I am sure you had no idea that the simple antacid tablet you were taking contained properties which could reduce the digestion and absorption of the food you eat.

That's right! That roll of antacid tablets which you probably have somewhere in your house at this very moment, when used properly—can help you lose weight and reduce your absorption of calories.

In addition, these tablets are more easily available, at less cost, and with fewer side-effects than any other weight-reduction aid I have ever encountered. When used on a temporary basis in conjunction with the Megatetic Program, these tablets will help you lose pounds and maintain your lowered weight more easily than you believed possible.

Since it is not my purpose to promote any particular brand of antacid, the following is a partial list of products which contain the necessary ingredients to be used as a Megatetic tablet:

Al - Caroid
Alkets
Amitone
Dicarbosil
Ratio
Titralac
Tums

Although there are many other brands of antacid available, the above list reflects those which contain the essential components. Use of an antacid not on the list may result in little or no benefit.

WHY ONE PATIENT LOST MORE THAN SHE WANTED

Norma W. was 28 years old, and although she weighed 157 pounds when she began on her Megatetic Program, she only needed to lose 23 pounds to reach her desirable weight. Halfway through her third week, Norma had achieved her final goal—ahead of schedule.

She therefore started on her post-program procedure which is necessary to maintain the lowered weight.

One week later, however, Norma had lost another six pounds. In this particular case the additional weight loss was not desired and therefore had to be reversed. I questioned Norma about her eating habits to see if I could find the reason she was continuing to lose weight. "I've been taking the tablets and eating the foods you recommended, but for some reason I'm just not as hungry as I used to be," Norma replied when I asked her about her eating habits. "What do you mean?" I asked.

"Well," she answered, "ever since I started on the post-program schedule, I just don't seem to eat as much as I did before. I'm not trying to limit the food I eat but I just don't seem to be hungry."

As I continued to question Norma, I found that she had been taking her tablets one-half hour before eating, and again immediately after finishing. Although she had been advised to take the tablets just before eating, she had interpreted this to mean some time prior to eating, and had therefore set up a schedule for herself. One-half hour before she knew she would be eating, she took two tablets. She did this before each meal. It took severals more days before I finally realized what was happening. By taking her tablets 30 minutes before meals Norma was initiating the digestive process. Apparently, the tablets stimulated the neurological mechanism responsible for digestion. Therefore, by the the time she sat down to eat, a portion of the digestive cycle had already been completed. Food did not produce new appetite and Norma thus ate less than permitted. Because of this she had continued to lose weight.

Once this was pointed out to her, Norma began taking her tablets immediately before eating. The weight loss diminished and gradually Norma maintained her proper level.

Since that time, I have experimented with timing the taking of the tablets. By adjusting the amount of time between tablets and food, I have been able to control, at least in part, the post-program weight maintenance or reduction in most patients.

HOW TO USE THE MEGATETIC TABLET
FOR CONTINUED SLENDERNESS

Although you can use the Megatetic tablet to lose weight as well as to maintain your lowered weight, it should only be used on a temporary basis. Reliance on any medication for long periods of time is contraindicated unless prescribed by a physician.

To maintain your lowered weight once you have completed your 30-day program all you need do is take two tablets (only one is necessary if you are using Alkets brand) five to ten minutes prior to eating. As soon as you finish eating, another two tablets should be taken (one Alket). Never take more than 16 tablets (8 if you are using Alkets) in 24 hours; nor continue taking the tablets for more than two weeks without at least a one week interruption. If you are concerned about some specific health problem or wish to exceed the above recommendations, please consult your family physician. Follow the post-program procedure as outlined in Chapter 11 relative to your food intake, and you will have no difficulty in maintaining your desirable weight.

Use of the Megatetic tablet will produce marvelous results. In Chapter 11, I present additional ways to use this tablet in conjunction with alternate approaches to weight reduction which I know you will enjoy.

INCREASING VITAMIN INTAKE FOR A HEALTHY PROGRAM

During your 30-day program the amount of nutrients you consume will be severely restricted. In order to preclude any adverse side-effects from your reduced intake of vitamins and minerals, you should take a nutrutional supplement.

Since there are dozens of well-known multi-vitamin preparations on the market, it is unnecessary for me to recommend a specific brand. Any multi-vitamin/mineral compound advised by your physician or pharmacist should be more than sufficient. Be sure that the label recommends only one tablet daily as a *supplement*. During the program you will be directed to take as many as three tablets in one 24-hour period. This is done so as to prevent any vitamin deficiency. If the multivitamin-mineral preparation you buy does not contain the recommended quantities of nutrients necessary to be used as a supplement, it will be too weak to prevent some minor deficiencies; if labeled *Therapeutic* dosage, it will be too strong, and may cause gastric distress. Be sure to purchase only those preparations which recommend *one tablet daily*. Also, follow the recommendations in Chapter 7, and you will not have to concern yourself about vitamin deficiency.

6 | HOW TO BURN UP CALORIES WITHOUT EXERCISE

Is there anything more depressing than having to perform routine and boring exercise programs? I doubt it! Most overweight patients detest weight lifting, calisthenics, jogging and most other physical activities. Personally, I feel that the overweight individual reacts to exercise programs in the same way most people respond to having to do something because "it is good for them." You, too, probably shun many physical activities for the same reason.

Once you attain a desirable weight, however, you will most likely take part in physical activities you enjoy. Swimming, tennis, skiing and all other active pastimes will hopefully become part of your new lifestyle. However, at that time you will be participating because you want to, and not because you have to. This, of course, is excellent not only from a physical, but from a psychological viewpoint. You will no longer feel foolish on the dance floor, nor ugly in a bathing suit. You will be happy and proud of your new slender physique. You will want to be part of the action and not just a spectator.

First, however, you must achieve that new, slender body. Since exercises are out, a different approach to increased utilization of calories must be available. This is the purpose of the *Energy Expender*.

HOW THE ENERGY EXPENDER WORKS

Every time you perform physical activity, whether it be brushing your teeth, polishing your shoes, or merely changing channels on the TV, numerous muscle groups throughout your body come into play. By means of a complex neurological mechanism initiated in the cortex of the brain, thousands upon thousands of individual muscle fibers are stimulated to contract each time you complete even the simplest tasks. With each contraction, energy in the form of calories is expended. It is in this way that exercise programs seek to increase your energy expenditure. If, however, you dislike programmed exercises, how will you expend increased amounts of energy? How will you use up those excess calories presently stored in the form of fat throughout your body? The answer, of course, is the Energy Expender. By incorporating the basic concepts of the Energy Expender system into your daily activities you will burn up hundreds and even thousands of extra calories without performing a single exercise.

Very simply stated, the Energy Expender is designed to produce increased caloric utilization without the need of prescribed exercise. This is accomplished by altering your daily activities in such a manner as to use up more calories than you normally would.

ALTERING YOUR ENVIRONMENT FOR WEIGHT LOSS

Each one of us lives in a unique environment. An environment specifically suited to our individual requirements. Every day, as we go about our chores, we continually alter this environment to some degree. This is usually done without much thought, and generally results in only minor changes in our daily energy expenditure.

By consciously and methodically altering your environment or surroundings, however, you can realize vastly increased energy expenditure.

Since your immediate environment is unique and coincides with your particular lifestyle, it will take some conscious effort on your part to make the necessary changes. Keep in mind that what you are trying to accomplish is a relatively new environment which will help you lose pounds. If properly designed, your new environment will also help you maintain a lowered weight level for the rest of your life.

In order to accomplish this, one simple rule should be remembered:

"Wherever you are, analyze the relationship of things about you."

For instance, if you are lying in bed, think about your relationship to:

1) reading light
2) night table
3) alarm clock
4) closets
5) chests and bureaus
6) doors and passageways
7) bathroom
8) chairs
9) clothing racks
10) etc.

Ask yourself the following questions:

"Can I move my bed so as to effect a new relationship to the things about me?"

"Can I rearrange other pieces of furniture to accomplish the same end?"

In the following illustrations I have attempted to show a before and after situation. In Figure #1 you will note that all items in the room bear a distinct efficient relationship to one another. In Figure #2 I have rearranged several of the items so as to produce surroundings which will assist in losing weight.

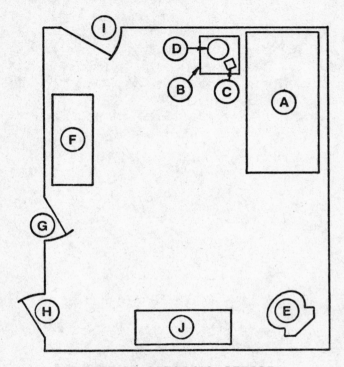

FIGURE 6-1: BEDROOM—BEFORE.

(A) Bed	(F) Chest of Drawers
(B) Nightstand	(G) Closet
(C) Alarm Clock	(H) Bath Access
(D) Lamp	(I) Hall Door
(E) Chair	(J) Table

In the above illustration all furniture has been placed so as to facilitate normal activities with the least amount of energy expenditure. The lamp (D), alarm clock (C) and nightstand (B) have been placed next to the bed (A) and are therefore easily accessible. The chest of drawers (F) is near the closet and bathroom to facilitate dressing.

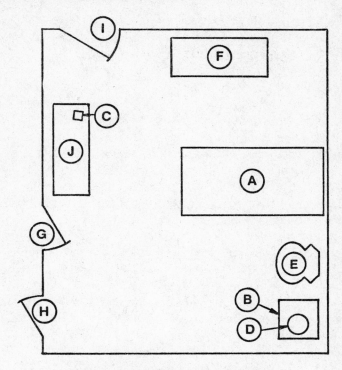

FIGURE 6-2: BEDROOM—AFTER.

Although the above illustration contains the same furniture as Figure # 1, certain rearrangements have been made. Since the most commonly occupied space is the bed (A), I have rearranged the furniture taking this into consideration. In this newly rearranged bedroom you would find it necessary to get out of bed to set or shut off the alarm clock (C). This is also true of the lamp (D). In addition, the lamp's placement would require use of the chair for reading (or smoking). The chest of drawers has been moved away from the closet. This results in extra steps when dressing. All in all this simple rearrangement of furniture would result in hundreds of extra calories being used up each week.

By duplicating similar rearrangements throughout your home you can burn up thousands of extra calories without exercises.

The above illustrations reveal very simply that a relatively small alteration can result in significant energy expenditure. In the particular case illustrated, the altered environment will result in an increased weekly usage in excess of *300* calories.

That's not bad when you consider that once you have made changes you no longer have to give it any thought. For as long as you use that particular room and its new environment, you will continue to burn up those extra calories every week.

By burning a similar number of calories in each room in your home, apartment or place of business, you will produce a situation which will continually work to keep you slender.

It is not necessary for you to make major alterations. One or two pieces of furniture in each room will do nicely. Don't overdo it, and don't be concerned with the exact number of calories which will be expended. Each day as you function in your altered environment you will consistently burn up extra calories, and that means extra pounds lost. In addition to the constant energy expenditure caused by your new surroundings, you will have also burned up considerable energy moving furniture about. You have, in effect, therefore, burned up a large initial number of calories and also produced a situation which will allow you to burn extra calories every day for the rest of your life. This is not dissimilar to the results obtained through a prescribed daily exercise program.

Remember,

>**"Wherever you are, analyze the relationship of things about you,"**

and you will lose extra pounds without exercise.

CHANGING METHODS TO CONTROL EFFICIENCY

In the same way that altering your environment increases energy expenditure, a change in methods will also produce greater weight loss. At the present time you are probably very efficient in the way you approach your daily chores. Although this is excellent, it tends to result in lessened energy expenditure with resultant obesity.

If you will make several minor changes in the way you do things, you will produce a greatly increased expenditure of energy.

With only a few changes this can result in hundreds, and even thousands, of extra calories burned each week.

If you are a housewife, the kitchen is probably the best place to make changes. By buying fresh foods as opposed to packaged ones you can burn up several hundred calories just preparing meals. Using a hand mixer instead of an electric one means additional calories burned. I am sure that if you analyzed your daily activities you could find literally dozens of ways to burn off those excess pounds. Major changes are not necessary, so don't overdo it.

For the individual who goes to business, method changing also works well. *Voluntarily* standing on the bus or train, walking up that last flight of stairs, or running your own small errands, can mean thousands of calories a week. The ways in which you can change your everyday activities are too numerous to mention. A little thought on your part will result in rapid and *sustained* weight loss. By using the Energy Expender guide at the end of this chapter you will be amazed at how quickly you burn off those excess pounds—all without routine exercises.

HOW PAULA T. MADE IT EASY

Paula T. was 36 years old and grossly overweight. She had been married for 13 years and had two school-age children. When I first saw her she was determined to lose those excess pounds and was willing to do almost anything to achieve success. Once I explained the Energy Expender system to her, Paula began to make numerous changes in her environment and methods.

Several weeks passed and Paula was losing weight faster than anticipated. On one of her visits to the Center I questioned Paula about her progress. As she related her story I realized that one of her method changes was primarily responsible for her rapid weight loss.

Prior to beginning on the Megatetic Program, Paula had done her family food shopping once a week. If for some reason she ran short of an item before her next trip to the market, she would call her husband and ask him to stop at the store and bring it home after work. All in all, Paula spent approximately 1½ hours per week doing her grocery shopping.

Once she began to make method changes, Paula T. realized

that one way she could increase her energy expenditure was to shop more often. She set up a schedule, and every day she would take a leisurely walk to the market. She would buy only enough food for that particular day. By doing this she found that she never ran short of an item and also that she could buy fresh produce without fear that it would spoil before her family could eat it. At the time of Paula's visit to me, she stated that she was spending more than 7 hours a week shopping. She reported that before going on the program those extra hours had been spent watching "soap operas." She further remarked that she enjoyed getting out of the house; seeing some of her friends; cooking what she knew was better food for her family; and generally being more active than previously.

When I asked Paula if she thought her method change was difficult or too much trouble, she simply replied, "No! It's easy." Paula went on to complete her program successfully. Final weight loss was 43 pounds.

LOSE EXTRA POUNDS BY (NOT) THINKING BEFORE DOING

Most overweight individuals, as has been stated previously, are very efficient. In addition to this, however, they also give considerable thought to each and every movement they make. When required to perform some specific task, they often consider what other tasks might be completed simultaneously. In this way they kill two (or more) birds with one stone. Usually this ability to perform several chores at once is beneficial. Oftentimes, however, when every chore must be thoroughly analyzed, you will find certain ones are not essential, or can be postponed. At the same time other duties can be relegated to another individual. In still additional cases a less strenuous method of accomplishing the task can be devised.

Sometimes the benefits accrued through intensive analysis are worthwhile, but in most cases the work to be done is minor, and could be completed before you even have time to consider various methods of performing it. This is the reason I advise you *not* to think before doing. I am not referring to important and complex decisions, but rather to simple, everyday chores such as making a particular telephone call, changing bed linens, starting a new hobby, painting the kitchen, etc.

Don't over-think! You will probably never do what you are thinking about. If something must be done—do it! Don't put it off and don't wait for someone else to do it.

YOUR ENERGY EXPENDER GUIDE

The following guide will assist you in formulating your own personal Energy Expender system. By permanently and continuously changing your surroundings and methods you will achieve a degree of energy expenditure comparable to vigorous and sustained exercise programs. Use your Expender as directed in Chapter 7 and you will never have to exercise again.

Environment Alteration

1. Visualize yourself in the most commonly occupied place in each room of your home or place of business.
2. Consider how you use each of the various items in that room (i.e., furniture, appliances, utensils, tools, equipment, etc.).
3. Formulate a furniture or item relocation program, keeping in mind that you want to expend more energy than at present.
4. Once you have initiated your alterations you should find that most activities performed in that particular room take considerably more time or expend more energy.
5. Re-evaluate your environment alteration. Try to find additional ways in which you can further increase your energy expenditure.

Method Change

1. Think about and write down a list of your daily activities. Try to set this up in chronological order as you would normally proceed through your day.

2. Analyze each activity and write down at least one way you can change it to produce increased energy expenditure.
3. If you have already altered your environment, many method changes will come about automatically. Additional changes should be made though, as this will greatly increase the number of calories you burn up each day.

Not Thinking

1. Train yourself to act.
2. Every time you realize something should be done, do it immediately.
3. Do not consider every possible alternative to action.
4. By doing more and analyzing less, much will be accomplished, including extra pounds lost.

A LIST OF 30 POSSIBLE SUGGESTIONS

Many of the following suggestions will be found in other chapters. They have been brought together here to assist you in setting up your personal Energy Expender system.

1. Get up ¼ hour earlier than usual (even on days off).
2. Get out on the wrong (opposite) side of the bed.
3. Be sure your alarm clock is placed as far from your bed as possible.
4. Shower at least once a day, but if possible try three times.
5. Shave every day. Even on days off.
6. Wash your hair several times weekly.
7. Brush teeth after *every* meal and before retiring.
8. Comb or brush your hair often.
9. Replace makeup at least one extra time each day.
10. Change bed linens at least twice a week.
11. Change clothes two, and if possible three, times daily.
12. Rearrange furniture frequently.

13. Relocate clothes in closets, bureaus, chests.
14. Re-arrange pots, pans, utensils, canned and bottled goods, dishes, plates, silverware, refrigerator and freezer shelves, storage and utility rooms.
15. Clean house more often.
16. Wax furniture at least twice a week.
17. Iron clothes even though you might get by without it.
18. Shop more often.
19. Walk don't ride.
20. Start a new hobby.
21. Take on extra work at the office.
22. Take a walk during coffee breaks and lunch hours.
23. Limit TV and reading time so as to increase activity time.
24. Clean and rearrange all tools.
25. Run your own errands.
26. Do those chores you've been putting off.
27. Vacuum every day.
28. Painting? Use a brush not a roller.
29. Get out in the garden.
30. Do more!!

. . . and you will definitely weigh less.

THE IMPORTANCE OF USING THE RIGHT ENERGY EXPENDERS

Donna was a beautiful young woman. She had first entered the Center seeking help for residual bursitis, but during the course of her therapy had made it known that she was also interested in losing a few pounds. Actually Donna was only eight pounds over her desirable weight and for a woman 24 years old didn't really appear in need of weight reduction. Nevertheless, Donna was adamant. She knew she was overweight and was determined to "knock off those extra pounds". When I discussed the Mini-Megatetic program with Donna, I learned that she had been slightly overweight ever since she could remember. Fortunately she had always been able to control her eating habits so as to preclude any major weight gain, but Donna felt she would be much happier if she could lose the few extra pounds she was carrying. She explained that she had little trouble in losing the weight (as she had done so several times in the past) but just couldn't seem to keep it off. It was therefore decided that the Mini-Megatetic program would be just right for Donna. In addition, I asked her to be overly conscientious about formulating her Energy Expenders. I wanted her to choose energy expending methods that would quickly become a part of her lifestyle and would therefore continue to benefit her after completion of the program. In the few short days it took Donna to complete her program she lost the required eight pounds but unfortunately I had placed too much emphasis on the Energy Expender. Donna had put together and initiated several methods of increasing her calorie utilization which, if continued, would have produced a gradual yet continuing weight loss. This, in and of itself, would have caused no great problem. The real problem was that most of the Energy Expenders Donna had chosen were of a temporary nature and would have required a continuous and conscious effort on her part. In a short time the Energy Expenders would have become distasteful and therefore discarded—with a resultant regaining of weight. I explained this to Donna and asked her to formulate a new set of Energy Expenders. The next day she returned and we discussed her ideas. Each and every Expender fit nicely into her lifestyle. It was easy to see that once she performed the activities for a week or two they would become a part of her. She would not have to consciously think about them nor force herself to do anything which was not natural for her.

The reason I have included this short case history is to dramatize the importance of choosing the proper Energy Expenders for you. Give careful consideration to the various methods of increasing your calorie utilization before deciding on which ones will best serve your purpose. For Donna, the following list of activities were just right:

1) Shower every morning upon awakening, and every evening upon returning from work.
2) Shampoo hair twice weekly, but wash hair with plain cool water each night to remove excess oils.

3) Set hair every night.
4) Brush teeth after each meal and before retiring. Use soft bristle brush and non-abrasive toothpaste.
5) Go bicycling for at least 30 minutes each evening before dinner.

THE INNOVATIVE ENERGY EXPENDER OF MIKE J.

Mike J. is a married man 44 years of age. He works at the County Courthouse some 20 miles from his home and has what is normally called a "desk-job".

Mike was quite active in sports as a young man but he no longer had the desire or the energy to take part in routine physical activities. It was this lack of energy which first brought Mike to the Center. He was concerned about it and thought it might be due to some blood disorder. Our examinations revealed a healthy middle-aged man some 20 pounds overweight. Although we recommended a weight loss program for Mike he was not really enthusiastic about it. Mike felt that he would do better on his own and therefore rejected any thought of following a prescribed regimen. Since he had originally come to the Center because of his chronic tiredness. Mike felt that if all he had to do was lose a few pounds, he would do it on his own. It should be noted here that Mike had never before tried to diet. His weight gain had been gradual, and had gone almost unnoticed. If we had not made the suggestion that Mike lose those extra pounds he probably never would have given his obesity a second thought. Nevertheless, several months later Mike returned to the Center. He had tried to lose those excess pounds but had been unsuccessful. He reported that he had reduced his weight several times only to regain it again. He felt as though he were on a see-saw—down one minute and up the next. He finally conceded that losing weight was only half the battle. Maintaining that lowered weight was the other half.

Since Mike seemed determined to overcome his weight problem, he was put on the Megatetic Program. He was fascinated by the completeness and specificity of the Megatetic approach and became extremely interested in the Energy Expender portion of the program. Needless to say, Mike was successful in reducing and maintaining his lowered weight. The Energy Expender which he formulated for his personal use incorporated almost every method which had been used up until that time. In addition, Mike sought out new ways to burn up calories. He no longer left his car in his driveway overnight. Instead, each evening he would pull it into his garage and close the garage door. This simple innovation resulted in a minimum of 28 garage door openings and closings weekly. When Mike went to work each morning he no longer parked in the Courthouse parking lot. Instead he would drive down two blocks to a municipal parking lot. Not only did this result in a four block walk each day but Mike also saved $1.35 a week in parking fees. On returning home each evening Mike took on a few extra chores. He began setting the dinner table and serving the meal. (His wife loved it!) In addition, Mike cleared the table after dinner, put left-overs away and did the dishes (by hand). Mike refused to watch TV before 9:00 pm; he began to cut his own lawn instead of having a neighbor's kid do it; he no longer brought his car to the car wash, but rather did it himself; he began helping his wife with housework; shined his shoes *every* morning; and in every possible way forced himself to be more active. By the time Mike completed his program he was at the proper weight and had energy to spare. The simple act of removing excess pounds along with a routine method of expending energy resulted in better physical and emotional health for Mike J. It could also do the same for you.

THE IMPORTANCE OF VARIOUS ACTIVITIES
ON ENERGY EXPENDITURE

The following list of activities is fairly complete. Since it is impossible to enumerate each and every physical action it will be necessary for you to substitute similar activities for those which appear on the list. For instance, the number of calories expended by typewriting rapidly would be very nearly the same as operating a computer console or using a keypunch or bookkeeping machine. As you proceed through your normal daily routine you will recognize activities which although not exactly the same as those listed, will be close enough to one or more activities to permit you to approximate the number of calories being expended.

Since each individual's basal metabolic rate (the rate at which you burn up calories) is different, the number of calories you expend with each activity will differ from those listed. The important thing though, is to recognize those activities which produce a greater expenditure of energy and to perform those activities more often during your regular day. By doing this you will increase the benefits of your Energy Expender program enormously and reduce your weight more rapidly.

In the post-program procedure, where the Energy Expender is used primarily for weight maintenance, you will find this list to be invaluable in assisting you to maintain a balance between calorie intake and expenditure.

ACTIVITY	CALORIES PER HOUR APPROXIMATE
Sleeping	65
Awake, Lying Still	77
Sitting Quietly	98
Eating	98
Reading Aloud	98
Sewing, Hand	98
Sewing, Electric Machine	98
Writing	98
Crocheting	99
Standing, Relaxed	105
Brushing Teeth	110
Paring Potatoes	112
Sewing, Foot Driven Machine	112
Standing, At Attention	112
Combing/Brushing Hair	112
Dressing and Undressing	119
Showering	120
Knitting a Sweater	122
Piano Playing, Slow	126

Singing, Loud	126
Preparing a Meal	130
Driving an Auto	133
Tailoring	135
Dishwashing	140
Ironing	140
Typewriting, Rapidly	140
Grocery Shopping	145
Washing, Car	148
Making Beds/Housecleaning	149
Washing Floors	154
Laundry, Light	161
Horseback Riding, Walk	168
Sweeping, With Broom	168
Light Exercise	170
Painting, Furniture	175
Sweeping, With Carpet Sweeper	182
Piano Playing, Fast	210
Walking 3 m.p.h.	210
Carpentry, Heavy	231
Bicycling, Moderate Speed	245
Vacuum Cleaning	259
Dancing, Waltz	280
Active Exercsise	290
Walking 4 m.p.h.	308
Skating	315
Dancing, Fast	336
Horseback Riding, Trot	371
Severe Exercise	450
Sawing Wood	480
Swimming, Leisurely	500
Running	560
Very Severe Exercise	600
Swimming, 2 m.p.h.	623
Walking, 5 m.p.h.	651
Walking, Up Stairs	1100

7 | YOUR MEGATETIC KIT

In previous chapters you have learned about the basic components of the Megatetic Weight Reduction Program. I am sure that by this time you are aware of why Megatetics is unique and why it is so successful. In this chapter, all of the various components are brought together for you in the form of a working kit.

As in any successful venture, the Megatetic Weight Reduction Program relies on proper organization, interim goals, and continued evaluation. Unlike most diets, however, the Megatetic Program allows you to keep abreast of your progress. Each day is planned and programmed just for you. You will never feel uncertain as to whether you are being successful or not. Each and every day you will mark and note your progress. You will know exactly how well you are doing and will be able to immediately alter your program as needed.

In this chapter you will find included nearly all the necessary materials for successfully completing your 30 days of rapid weight loss. The only additional item you will need will be a standard calendar. It should be large enough so that you will be able to note your progress and indicate the activities and directions completed on schedule. A good calendar for this purpose is the common "calendar pad" which shows one day on each page. This type can be obtained at any stationery store, but it is not essential. Any large calendar, or a notebook with the days filled in, will suffice. Use these materials—and you too will be pleased and excited about the results. Don't allow yourself to become sidetracked, and be sure to proceed according to plan . . . in just 30 days you won't believe your own slenderness.

PREPARING YOURSELF FOR SLENDERNESS

Most overweight individuals want to lose weight desperately. They feel self-conscious about their size and are often unhappy. Unfortunately, when they attempt to lose those unwanted pounds they rarely have a long-range plan or final goal in mind. They begin on some crash program without giving adequate thought to their ultimate goal. Usually, within a few days they have lost their motivation. Their initial excitement wears off and they gradually lose track of their dietary program. It is, therefore, essential to have a clear-cut view of your ultimate goals. Although your total weight loss is of primary importance, you should also have in view some visual goals.

USING VISUAL GOALS TO ACHIEVE RAPID WEIGHT LOSS

Magazines are probably the best source of visual goal images. Photographs depicting what *you* want to look like, and of what *you* want to accomplish, are excellent reminders of your visual goal image. Take a few hours when starting on your Megatetic Weight Reduction Program and find several photographs of people with bodies similar to what you want to achieve (See DAY 1, page 109). Perhaps you can already visualize yourself wearing certain types of clothing, such as bikinis or shorts. Find pictures that reflect this, that coincide with your goals, and cut them out. Some individuals are activity oriented. They would like to be able to do certain things, take part in certain activities. If this is the case with you, find

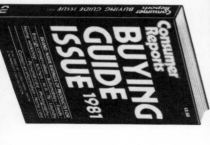

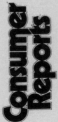

pictures of people performing those activities and clip them out. One picture which depicts your ideal, dressed in desirable clothing and performing acitvities which you would like to perform, is worth more than all the continued warnings and self-recriminations you have heard or spoken, about being overweight.

You should have at least five different visual images in the form of clippings or photographs when starting on your weight reduction program. They can be of people, clothes, activities, or combinations of these. It will then be easier for you to visualize your final goal and to keep its desirability in focus throughout your 30-day program.

FOUR IDEAS OTHERS HAVE USED TO STAY ON THE TRACK TO SLENDERNESS

1. *Thelma A.* had completed her Megatetic Weight Reduction Program successfully. She had reached her first interim goal ahead of schedule and had lost the desired amount of weight during the 30-day period. In re-evaluating her progress, I noted that at one point prior to reaching her second interim goal, Thelma's weight loss had come to a standstill. When I asked her about this, Thelma explained that because she lost weight so quickly in the beginning, she had lost some of her motivation. She thought that since she was doing so well she didn't have to pay strict attention to the program and had started "cheating". Only after not meeting her second goal did she realize that she had better get down to business. She found some pictures of grossly overweight people, who had allowed themselves to become grotesque because of their extreme heaviness. She placed these pictures in strategic locations around her home. She explained, that for her it wasn't enough to just want to look like her ideals. When she saw what she could become if she didn't pay attention to the program, she made up her mind to no longer "cheat". Apparently, Thelma realized that it wasn't only her desire to achieve her final goal but also her dislike of what she had been and could become again, that helped her get back on the track.

2. *Kathy M.* was twenty-two years of age. She had gained

considerable weight since her marriage some two years prior. During one of our consultations, after Kathy had been successful on her program, she told me about her method of increasing her motivation.

During her second week on the program Kathy realized that her husband's birthday was coming up and that she really wanted to look good for that occasion. She went out and bought an outfit that she knew she could wear only if she lost the necessary pounds. Every day she tried to get into the new clothes; and every day she realized she was getting closer. On the 27th day of her program she was successful. The new clothes fit her and she modeled them for her husband the following week. For Kathy, her desire to please her husband as well as herself was all the motivation she needed.

I have given this idea to other patients and have found it helps many. Whether birthday, holiday, social function, anniversary, or whatever; making a reasonable commitment by buying some clothing that won't fit unless you achieve your goal, really works.

3. *Louise C.* seemed to be failing on her program. She had lost some weight initially, but now seemed to have "plateaued out". She was maintaining her overweight condition. When asked about this, Louise admitted that she was "snackin' ". Even the photograph on the door of the refrigerator (her visual goal) wasn't stopping her from eating. In an effort to help, I suggested that she put her bathroom scale in front of the refrigerator door. It worked! Every time Louise started to get a snack, she had to move the scale. Instead, she would get on it and see how well she was doing. Her "snackin' " stopped and Louise continued to meet her goals.

4. *Barbara K.* was 24 years old. After being successful on her Megatetic Weight Reduction Program, Barbara told me that one of the pictures she had originally chosen for her goal purposes showed young men and women yachting. She confessed that after she chose this picture, she also made up a complete fantasy about it, and put herself in the place of one of the girls in the photograph. For 30 days she lived the fantasy! Every day she saw herself as beautiful and desirable, and enjoying herself while yachting. Today Barbara *is* beautiful and enjoying many outdoor activities including yachting. She is very popular and always has dates.

DETERMINING HOW MANY POUNDS
YOU WANT TO LOSE

In addition to visual images, you will also benefit from setting up interim and final goals regarding your desired weight loss. Use Chart A or B, Chart of Desirable Weights to determine what weight you want to be at the end of your 30-day program. Then, subtract this desired weight from your starting weight (See DAY 1) to determine your final weight-loss goal.*

Once you have determined your final weight-loss goal (viz., the number of pounds you want to lose during your 30-day program) you will be able to find your interim weight-loss goals on Chart C. These interim goals represent the number of pounds you

CHART A:
DESIRABLE WEIGHT FOR MEN WHO
ARE PRESENTLY OVERWEIGHT
(See DAY 1 For Starting Weight)

Height	Small Frame	Medium Frame	Large Frame
5'2"	118-125	123-135	132-149
5'3"	121-129	127-138	135-151
5'4"	125-133	130-143	138-156
5'5"	129-136	135-147	142-160
5'6"	132-142	137-153	146-167
5'7"	135-145	143-157	150-170
5'8"	140-150	146-161	155-175
5'9"	144-153	150-165	160-180
5'10"	148-158	154-170	164-185
5'11"	153-163	157-174	168-189
6'0"	156-167	162-180	173-194
6'1"	161-171	167-185	178-199
6'2"	163-174	173-191	183-204
6'3"	167-177	178-199	189-216
6'4"	171-180	187-205	196-225

*If your final weight-loss goal exceeds 50 pounds, you should not try to lose the full amount in one 30-day period. Rather, you should divide the total weight loss desired into equal parts of less than 50 pounds and then proceed with one 30-day program at a time until your total weight loss is achieved.

CHART B:
DESIRABLE WEIGHT FOR WOMEN WHO
ARE PRESENTLY OVERWEIGHT
(See DAY 1 For Starting Weight)

Height	Small Frame	Medium Frame	Large Frame
4'10"	93-99	98-111	106-123
4'11"	96-104	101-114	108-126
5'0"	98-108	104-116	113-129
5'1"	103-111	107-119	115-132
5'2"	105-114	111-123	119-135
5'3"	108-116	113-125	121-138
5'4"	111-119	116-130	125-142
5'5"	115-123	120-134	129-147
5'6"	117-127	125-140	134-151
5'7"	122-131	128-143	137-154
5'8"	125-135	132-148	141-158
5'9"	130-140	136-151	145-163
5'10"	133-143	140-156	149-168
5'11"	138-149	145-159	153-175
6'0"	142-154	150-164	158-180

CHART C: INTERIM GOALS
Final Weight Loss Desired

	5*	10*	15	20	25	30	35	40	45	50
1st Goal Day 6	5	10	12	14	15	18	19	20	22	24
2nd Goal Day 11			15	17	19	21	23	25	27	28
3rd Goal Day 14				20	22	24	26	29	31	35
4th Goal Day 21					25	27	29	33	38	43
5th Goal Day 25						30	33	38	43	48
6th Goal Day 30							35	40	45	50

should lose at various times during the program. By using these interim goals you will find it much easier to achieve continuous and

---

* If 10 or fewer pounds is all you must lose, the full 30-day program may produce too much weight loss. See Chapter 8 for specific recommendations.

rapid weight loss. If, however, you require a weight loss of 10 pounds or less, follow directions in Chapter 8 and eliminate all interim goal determinations.

Find your final weight-loss goal on the top line of Chart C. By reading down you will be able to determine your interim goals (See DAY 1).

KEEPING YOUR WEIGHT LOSS ON SCHEDULE

In any dietary program, keeping yourself on schedule is probably the most important factor. If you allow yourself to get away from what is most important, losing those extra pounds on schedule, you will find yourself not only discouraged, but it will also take enormous resolve to get back on the track. Each day of the Megatetic Weight Reduction Program is designed just for you. Be sure to use it as it was intended. Every day consult your Daily Schedule. Fill in the appropriate material and make notes or comments which you feel are important. There are six interim goals during your 30-day program. If for any reason you don't achieve a specific goal on the designated day, don't be discouraged. A few of my patients report that at least one interim goal was not met on schedule. This is due to the physiological differences of each individual and it can be expected in certain instances. If this happens to you, go back one day on your schedule. Prepare yourself for that particular interim goal one extra day. You will find that this extra preparation will put you back on schedule and you will then reach your interim goal as planned.

A very small number of patients have reported that they never achieved any of their goals on schedule, but, after long consultations it was found that they had cheated on their program in one way or another. Either they weren't following the dietary portion exactly; hadn't really changed their environment to any great extent; or "forgot" to take their Megatetic tablet. Once this was shown to them, they returned to their program and subsequently met or exceeded their goals.

In any event, you should never proceed with your program unless you achieve your specific goals as planned.

USING YOUR 30 DAILY SCHEDULES

On the following pages you will find your 30 individual Daily Schedules. Read and follow the instructions they contain, and in one short month you will achieve a greater weight loss than you ever thought possible.

The Megatetic Weight Reduction Program should be started on a Friday, as past experience has shown this to be best. Once again, follow the instructions and complete the necessary information as directed and you will be astonished at how rapidly you lose those pounds. On the calendar which you have obtained for this purpose, write down the information indicated on the Daily Schedules (This is an excellent activity for your first evening on the Megatetic Program).

AN ADDITIONAL SUGGESTION THAT LEADS TO SUCCESSFUL WEIGHT REDUCTION

One of the most beneficial points of the Megatetic Program is its "one day at a time" approach to weight reduction. Each day is planned and programmed for you—one day at a time. When you first start your 30-day program you need only fill in the information (as directed) on your daily calendar sheets, but it is strongly recommended that you not read the summary information or other data contained on upcoming Daily Schedules. Read, understand, and follow the recommendations TODAY—do not skip ahead through the Daily Schedules as this will only serve to confuse you and make your program appear more difficult than it really is.

Follow your Megatetic Program step by step, day by day, and in only a short time you will be slender.

DAILY SCHEDULE

FRIDAY

DAY 1

5 Days to First Interim Goal   Starting Weight   Lbs.

Less Desired Weight   Lbs.

Equals Final Weight Loss Goal   Lbs.

SUMMARY: Today is the beginning of your 30-day rapid weight-loss program. Eat breakfast and lunch as usual, but be sure that you don't overdo it. After lunch take no solid food, and drink nothing but water. This evening you may feel a slight weakness when it is time for dinner. This is not uncommon and is usually due to a lowering of your blood sugar. Weigh yourself at 6 PM this evening and record the weight on your calendar. This will be your starting weight for the purposes of the program.

Use this starting weight to determine your final and interim goals (pages 105 and 106) and write these goals in on the appropriate days of your calendar.

This evening, find and clip several visual goals, (page 102) and place them in strategic locations around your home, car, or wherever they will be helpful reminders.

0   Megatetic Tablet Prior to Breakfast (Chapter 5, p. 76)
00 Nutritional Supplements (Chapter 5, p. 79)
0   Megatetic Tablet Prior to Lunch
0   Starting Weight Determined
0   Final Goal Determined
0   Interim Goals Determined and Filled In
0   Visual Goals Clipped and Placed
0   Chart Started (page 140)

DAILY SCHEDULE

SATURDAY

DAY 2

4 Days to First Interim Goal
Starting Weight   Lbs.
Less Weight This AM Lbs.
Equals Weight Loss   Lbs.

SUMMARY: This morning your weight should be the same or slightly less than your starting weight. Some individuals even notice a slight gain. This is not uncommon so don't be concerned about it.

Today will be your first day of fasting. Take it easy and don't over exert yourself—water only today! Although you are not eating, you may still have a bowel movement. This is due to the residue still in the digestive tract. You may note some mid-day weariness and possibly some abdominal cramps. Your intestinal tract has not yet adapted to the fast. Headaches are not uncommon either. Their severity will depend on the degree of your previous overindulgence or overweight. This is a sign that your body is beginning to purify itself by ridding itself of toxic build up. If headaches persist, lie down and rest. Drink plenty of water, at least two quarts. This evening make a list of your daily activities (page 141). Then write down at least seven ways you will alter your environment to help expend increased amounts of energy. (See suggestions on page 143).

0 List of Daily Activities (page 141)
000000000 Glasses of Water Consumed
0 Chart Updated
0 Seven Ways to Increase Energy Expenditure

DAILY SCHEDULE

SUNDAY

DAY 3

3 Days to First Interim Goal

Starting Weight   Lbs.

Less Weight This AM   Lbs.

Equals Weight Loss   Lbs.

SUMMARY: This morning's weight should be much lower than yesterday. Several pounds is not uncommon and you will feel less bloated. Your body is ridding itself of unnecessary fluids and this is what causes the great loss of weight. Today you may feel tired. This is due to the increased toxin levels of the bloodstream as your body continues its "housecleaning". Cramps should subside and any headache should be slight although constant. You may note a coating of your tongue and notice a disagreeable mouth odor. This too is due to toxin excretion and is to be expected.

Today you will prepare to activate your Energy Expender by making any changes in your environment necessary to accommo date it. Water only and at least nine glasses.

0   Changed Environment in Preparation for Energy Expender

000000000   Glasses of Water Consumed

0   Chart Updated

DAILY SCHEDULE

MONDAY

DAY 4

2 Days to First Interim Goal   Starting Weight   Lbs.
                                                Less Weight This AM   Lbs.
                                                Equals Weight Loss   Lbs.

SUMMARY: This morning you should notice another loss of
weight. Probably not as large as yesterday. Mouth odor and coated
tongue should definitely be present. If not, your body is extremely
toxic and reversal will take longer. Moderate activity is indicated
although you still may feel tired. Be sure to initiate your Energy
Expender by incorporating at least one of your ideas from the list
into your daily routine. Your urine should be more concentrated.
Bowel movements may still be continuing, although in much smaller quantities.

0   Energy Expender Initiated
000000000   Glasses of Water Consumed
0   Chart Updated

DAILY SCHEDULE

TUESDAY

DAY 5

1 Day to First Interim Goal   Starting Weight   Lbs.

Less Weight This AM   Lbs.

Equals Weight Loss   Lbs.

SUMMARY: This morning's weight may be unchanged from yesterday or a slight reduction may be noticed. This indicates that the body has released as much unnecessary fluid as required and will now begin digesting its own fat. The digestive system is no longer active and some residual acid flow in the stomach may result in heartburn. Drink plenty of water to flush the system and relieve any gastric distress. Your tongue may start to clear and return to its normal pinkish color. This is a good sign. Be sure to add at least one more Energy Expender from your list to your daily routine.

Tomorrow is your first interim goal and you will have reached your first plateau. Your clothes are beginning to feel loose. Remember how it felt to have to squeeze into your clothing?

00 Energy Expenders Initiated

000000000 Glasses of Water Consumed

0 Chart Updated

DAILY SCHEDULE

WEDNESDAY

DAY 6

		Starting Weight	Lbs.
		Less Weight This AM	Lbs.
First Interim Goal	Lbs.	Equals Weight Loss	Lbs.

SUMMARY: You have reached your first interim goal. Congratulations! Your weight has dropped again, although only slightly. Another sign that your body is burning up its excess fat. You should feel much better today, as energy returns. You may (if desired) have three glasses (8 ounces each) of fruit or vegetable juices of your choice. Be sure that you mix equal amounts of juice (4 ounces) and water (4 ounces) before drinking. Otherwise the concentrated juice will cause acid rebound and/or stimulate a craving for food. Sip don't gulp! It should take at least 15 minutes to finish each glass of juice.

Be careful not to overdo it—today you may find it difficult to control your appetite. Be sure to drink sufficient amounts of water in addition to the juice. Don't lose sight of your ultimate goal, nor jeopardize your slenderness just for a shortlived gluttonous gorging. Don't forget to add another Expender today.

000   Glasses of Juice/Water Consumed
000000000   Glasses of Water Consumed
000   Energy Expenders Initiated
0   Chart Updated
000   Nutritional Supplements

DAILY SCHEDULE

THURSDAY

DAY 7

4 Days to Second Interim Goal   Starting Weight   Lbs.

Less Weight This AM   Lbs.

Equals Weight Loss   Lbs.

SUMMARY: Today you are back on your fast. Water only! Your weight today should show a slight gain over yesterday or at best a maintenance at the same weight. This is due to fluid retention from your juice drinking. You are on your way to your second interim goal. Today you may feel weak again due to sugar level alterations—ignore it—it will soon pass. You may be bothered by diarrhea. This too is not uncommon and indicates your body is still cleaning out its systems. Today is a good time to think about your final achievement; especially in terms of new clothing and activities. Have you bought yourself anything to wear for that special occasion? Continue on with your three Expenders.

000   Energy Expenders Initiated

000000000   Glasses of Water Consumed

0   Have You Considered New Clothes for That Special Occasion (page 104)

0   Chart Updated

DAILY SCHEDULE

FRIDAY

DAY 8

3 Days to Second Interim Goal   Starting Weight   Lbs.

Less Weight This AM   Lbs.

Equals Weight Loss   Lbs.

SUMMARY: It's the end of the week and you have lost more weight. By Monday your clothes will look baggy on you. Diarrhea may continue but shouldn't cause any major discomfort. Your tongue may have some slight coating. Tiredness is common but will disappear tomorrow. Add another Energy Expender to your schedule. It should be fairly easy going this weekend with your second interim goal just around the corner. At this point you should be able to more clearly visualize your final goals.

0000   Energy Expenders
000000000   Glasses of Water Consumed
0   Chart Updated

DAILY SCHEDULE

SATURDAY

DAY 9

2 Days to Second Interim Goal

Starting Weight   Lbs.
Less Weight This AM   Lbs.
Equals Weight Loss   Lbs.

SUMMARY: More weight lost. Only two more days of fasting and you will be at your second interim goal. You should feel quite good today. You should have five energy expenders incorporated in your daily schedule by this evening. Since energy should be returning today, you might consider some project around the house that you have been postponing. At this point in the program most patients report a mild euphoria associated with their increased energy levels.

0000   Energy Expenders Initiated
000000000   Glasses of Water Consumed
0   Chart Updated

DAILY SCHEDULE

SUNDAY

DAY 10

1 Day to Second Interim Goal   Starting Weight   Lbs.
                                     Less Weight This AM   Lbs.
                                     Equals Weight Loss   Lbs.

SUMMARY: Again, your weight is reduced. Although it might only be a slight reduction. Tomorrow your second interim goal day. You had better start thinking about new clothes—the ones you were wearing will no longer fit. It is just as important not to wear clothes that are too loose as it is to not wear tight fitting clothing. Today's newspaper is a good place to check for clothing sales. You should feel quite energetic and your tongue should be clear. Add another Expender to your schedule.

000000 Energy Expenders Initiated
000000000 Glasses of Water
0 Chart Updated

DAILY SCHEDULE

MONDAY

DAY 11

		Starting Weight	Lbs.
		Less Weight This AM	Lbs.
Second Interim Goal	Lbs.	Equals Weight Loss	Lbs.

SUMMARY: You have done it again! Meeting your Second Interim Goal indicates not only weight lost, but major reduction in your size. You must get new clothes that fit properly. Compliments are the password. Everyone has noticed a change. Be proud of it— today you will begin to take fluids in addition to water. The same as on Day 6. Juice mixed with water, only. No solid food of any kind. Your blood sugar level will increase. You will be quite energetic but may also feel bloated. Diarrhea is a possibility. Are there any Energy Expenders you might have overlooked? The extra calories they burn are needed for rapid weight loss.

000   Glasses of Juice/Water Consumed
000000000   Glasses of Water Consumed
000000   Energy Expenders Initiated
0   Additional Energy Expender?
0   Chart Updated
000   Nutritional Supplements

DAILY SCHEDULE

TUESDAY

DAY 12

2 Days to Third Interim Goal   Starting Weight   Lbs.
                                    Less Weight This AM   Lbs.
                                    Equals Weight Loss   Lbs.

SUMMARY: Have you gained some weight? Don't worry. This is
not unusual. However, you should still be able to notice a continuing reduction in size. Today you are on fluids again (same as yesterday). Energy levels are good. Two more days until Interim Goal
No. 3. Continue with your Energy Expenders and increase them if
possible. Everyone you meet should be remarking about how much
weight you've lost. Your motivation should be increased by these
compliments.

000   Glasses of Juice/Water Consumed
000000000   Glasses of Water Consumed
000000   Energy Expenders Initiated
0   Additional Energy Expender?
0   Chart Updated
000   Nutritional Supplements

DAILY SCHEDULE

WEDNESDAY

DAY 13

1 Day to Third Interim Goal   Starting Weight   Lbs.

Less Weight This AM   Lbs.

Equals Weight Loss   Lbs.

SUMMARY: Weight should be the same as yesterday or slightly reduced. Juices again today. Tomorrow is Interim Goal No. 3. Bowel movements increasing. Don't touch solid food. Have you changed your visual goals? At the start of your program you mentally visualized yourself on Day 30—if this image has changed— change your visual goals to coincide with it.

000   Glasses of Juice/Water Consumed

000000000   Glasses of Water Consumed

000000   Energy Expenders Initiated

0   Additional Energy Expender?

0   New Visual Goals?

0   Chart Updated

000   Nutritional Supplements

DAILY SCHEDULE

THURSDAY

DAY 14

		Starting Weight	Lbs.
		Less Weight This AM	Lbs.
Third Interim Goal	Lbs.	Equals Weight Loss	Lbs.

SUMMARY: Weight reduced again—your third goal achieved. Compliments continuing. Juices today—tomorrow is your last day of juices only—don't make any major alterations in type or quantity of fluids. With your first three goals achieved, your chart should look impressive. The major portions of weight have been lost and there should be a dramatic change in your appearance. Your next goal will be easier to achieve. Don't let your guard down. Friends will be coaxing you to "cheat".

000 Glasses of Juice/Water Consumed
000000000 Glasses of Water Consumed
000000 Energy Expenders Initiated
0 Additional Energy Expender?
0 Chart Updated
000 Nutritional Supplements

DAILY SCHEDULE

FRIDAY

DAY 15

6 Days to Fourth Interim Goal   Starting Weight   Lbs.
                                       Less Weight This AM   Lbs.
                                       Equals Weight Loss   Lbs.

SUMMARY: The weekend starts tomorrow and today you have lost more weight. Excess fat continues to melt from your body. Energy levels may be slightly decreased. This can be expected. If you bought new clothes last week, they probably are getting loose on you. No reason to buy anymore though, unless they will fit properly on Day 30. You will still lose considerable size over the next portion of your program. Energy Expenders should be habitual by now. This evening you might consider some additional new Expenders which will help you lose even faster.

000   Glasses of Juice/Water Consumed
000000000   Glasses of Water Consumed
000000   Energy Expenders Initiated
00   Additional Expenders?
0   Chart Updated
000   Nutritional Supplements

DAILY SCHEDULE

SATURDAY

DAY 16

5 Days to Fourth Interim Goal   Starting Weight   Lbs.

Less Weight This AM   Lbs.

Equals Weight Loss   Lbs.

SUMMARY: More pounds gone—today starts your third phase of the program. Three glasses of juice along with as much water as desired. Also, today you should add one piece of fruit to your intake. An apple is recommended, and I suggest you not eat it until the evening. Be careful! Chew the food until it is almost dissolved. Do not swallow large chunks as this might cause gastric distress Your body must slowly get used to processing solids again. Under no circumstances have more than one piece of fruit and be sure to take the Megatetic tablet before eating it. (Chapter 5, page 76) Keep busy so as not to fall into the trap of allowing your appetite to take over. Don't jeopardize all your success just for short-lived satisfaction.

000   Glasses of Juice/Water Consumed
000000000   Glasses of Water Consumed
0   Fruit Consumed
000000   Energy Expenders Initiated
00   Additional Energy Expenders?
0   Megatetic Tablet Prior to Solid Food
000   Nutritional Supplements
0   Chart Updated

DAILY SCHEDULE

SUNDAY

DAY 17

4 Days to Fourth Interim Goal   Starting Weight   Lbs.

Less Weight This AM   Lbs.

Equals Weight Loss   Lbs.

SUMMARY: Weight gain— no problem if slight and you didn't give in by eating more than you were supposed to. Today's intake is the same as yesterday. Juices and one piece of fruit. Chew well— slowly—diarrhea isn't uncommon today, but shouldn't cause any problem. Tomorrow should show additional weight loss. Energy levels are up today. You should add new methods of expending those calories.

000   Glasses of Juice/Water Consumed
000000000   Glasses of Water Consumed
0   Fruit Consumed
000000   Energy Expenders Initiated
00   Additional Energy Expenders?
0   Megatetic Tablet
000   Nutritional Supplements
0   Chart Updated

DAILY SCHEDULE

MONDAY

DAY 18

3 Days to Fourth Interim Goal   Starting Weight   Lbs.

Less Weight This AM   Lbs.

Equals Weight Loss   Lbs.

SUMMARY: You are definitely progressing. Weight loss may be slight but your size continues to go down. People are amazed at how quickly you have dropped your weight. Juices and fruit today. As before, you should eat the fruit in the evening. There may be some tiredness today—don't give in to it. Continue with your energy expenders and try to do more than usual. In less than two weeks you will be on a normal diet *and* be slender.

000   Glasses of Juice/Water Consumed
000000000   Glasses of Water Consumed
0   Fruit Consumed
000000   Energy Expenders Initiated
00   Additional Energy Expenders?
0   Megatetic Tablet
000   Nutritional Supplement
0   Chart Updated

DAILY SCHEDULE

TUESDAY

DAY 19

2 Days to Fourth Interim Goal   Starting Weight   Lbs.

Less Weight This AM   Lbs.

Equals Weight Loss   Lbs.

SUMMARY: Again the scale registers less. You should be feeling fine although bowel movements haven't stabilized. Juices and fruit as before. Are you continuing to increase your energy expenditure? Make plans for new activities—you won't be embarrassed by your overweight much longer. Your third week on the program is almost complete.

000   Glasses of Juice/Water Consumed

000000000   Glasses of Water Consumed

0   Fruit Consumed

000000   Energy Expenders Initiated

000   Additional Expenders?

0   Megatetic Tablet

000   Nutritional Supplements

0   Chart Updated

DAILY SCHEDULE

WEDNESDAY

DAY 20

1 Day to Fourth Interim Goal   Starting Weight   Lbs.
                                   Less Weight This AM   Lbs.
                                   Equals Weight Loss   Lbs.

SUMMARY: Mid-week and more weight lost—energy is up and
tomorrow is your next Interim Goal. Continue the same as yesterday. You should be checking on clothing sales because even your
new clothing hangs on you like so much burlap. Think positive—a
new wardrobe is waiting! Has anyone asked how you are losing
weight so fast? It takes years to put all those excess pounds on and
yet look how quickly they are melting away.

000 Glasses of Juice/Water Consumed
000000000 Glasses of Water Consumed
0 Fruit Consumed
000000 Energy Expenders Initiated
000 Additional Expenders?
0 Megatetic Tablet
000 Nutritional Supplements
0 Chart Updated

DAILY SCHEDULE

THURSDAY

DAY 21

		Starting Weight	Lbs.
		Less Weight This AM	Lbs.
Fourth Interim Goal	Lbs.	Equals Weight Loss	Lbs.

SUMMARY: Interim goal—can you believe how many pounds you have lost in just under three weeks? Today you will increase your intake to two pieces of fruit (two apples are suggested) along with juices. Continue to savor the solid food slowly, so as not to stimulate your appetite—chew the food until extremely fine. The increase in solid food may result in some gas and bloating. This is not uncommon so don't be concerned about it.

000 Glasses of Juice/Water Consumed
000000000 Glasses of Water Consumed
00 Fruit Consumed
000000 Energy Expenditures Initiated
000 Additional Expenders?
00 Megatetic Tablets
000 Nutritional Supplements
0 Chart Updated

DAILY SCHEDULE

FRIDAY

DAY 22

3 Days to Fifth Interim Goal   Starting Weight   Lbs.

Less Weight This AM   Lbs.

Equals Weight Loss   Lbs.

SUMMARY: Did you gain a pound or two? No problem, it is the residue build-up in the bowels. Tomorrow calls for another change in food intake—but today eat the same as yesterday. Be sure to take the Megatetic Tablets as directed. They are extremely important in the overall program. Some watery bowel movements can be expected today.

000   Glasses of Juice/Water Consumed

000000000   Glasses of Water Consumed

00   Fruit Consumed

000000   Energy Expenders Initiated

000   Additional Expenders?

00   Megatetic Tablets

000   Nutritional Supplements

0   Chart Updated

DAILY SCHEDULE

SATURDAY

DAY 23

2 Days to Fifth Interim Goal

Starting Weight   Lbs.
Less Weight This AM   Lbs.
Equals Weight Loss   Lbs.

SUMMARY: You may have gained slightly or lost a small amount
of weight depending on your digestive system. But no matter—
today your intake increases. Three juices, two fruits, and a salad.
The salad should be your evening meal. Mix up some lettuce, celery, and onion (if desired). Slice up a sour pickle and add it. No
dressing or salt though. It will still taste delicious. Be careful! Don't
overfill your dish—if you eat too much you will be sorry—not only
because you won't reach your next goal, but also because you will
feel miserable and bloated. At this point some patients overstuff
themselves because they remember the large portions they used to
eat. Don't be deceived! Eat a *small* salad—it will be satisfying.

000   Glasses of Juice/Water Consumed
000000000   Glasses of Water Consumed
00   Fruit Consumed
0   Salad Consumed
000000   Energy Expenders Initiated
000   Additional Expenders?
000   Megatetic Talbets
000   Nutritional Supplements
0   Chart Updated

DAILY SCHEDULE

SUNDAY

DAY 24

1 Day to Fifth Interim Goal   Starting Weight   Lbs.
                                     Less Weight This AM   Lbs.
                                    Equals Weight Loss   Lbs.

SUMMARY: Your weight has gone up in all probability. But you
continue to lose inches as your body uses up that excess fat. You
probably feel somewhat bloated and your bowels are active. Some
gas is common. With less than a week to go your body is making the
necessary alterations. Today your intake is the same as yesterday,
but your salad should, if anything, be smaller than last night's.

000   Glasses of Juice /Water Consumed
000000000   Glasses of Water Consumed
00   Fruit Consumed
0   Salad Consumed
000000   Energy Expenders Initiated
000   Additional Expenders?
000   Megatetic Tablets
000   Nutritional Supplements
0   Chart Updated

DAILY SCHEDULE
MONDAY
DAY 25

	Starting Weight	Lbs.
	Less Weight This AM	Lbs.
Fifth Interim Goal Lbs.	Equals Weight Loss	Lbs.

SUMMARY: A weight drop is usual this morning, although not necessary. Inches continue to melt away. You are at your next goal. Today you must eat two salads (small) but only one piece of fruit. Three glasses of watered juice are O.K. With only a few days left you should start picking out your new wardrobe. A commitment to continued slenderness is indicated.

000   Glasses Juice/Water Consumed
000000000   Glasses Water Consumed
0   Fruit Consumed
00   Salads Consumed
000000   Energy Expenders Initiated
000   Additional Expenders?
000   Megatetic Tablets
000   Nutritional Supplements
0   Chart Updated

DAILY SCHEDULE

TUESDAY

DAY 26

4 Days to Final Goal   Starting Weight   Lbs.
                                       Less Weight This AM   Lbs.
                                       Equals Weight Loss   Lbs.

SUMMARY: More weight and more inches lost. Today your intake
is the same as yesterday. Only a few days left so don't let anyone
dissuade you from your goal. You are on your way to your final goal
and it's only four days away.

000 Glasses Juice/Water Consumed
000000000 Glasses Water Consumed
0 Fruit Consumed
00 Salads Consumed
000000 Energy Expenders Initiated
000 Additional Expenders?
000 Megatetic Tablets
000 Nutritional Supplements
0 Chart Updated

DAILY SCHEDULE
WEDNESDAY
DAY 27

3 Days to Final Goal

	Starting Weight	Lbs.
	Less Weight This AM	Lbs.
	Equals Weight Loss	Lbs.

SUMMARY: You may not have lost any weight this morning, but this is common. However, your clothing should continue to feel larger on you. This morning you have a piece of fruit for breakfast, lunch is a small salad and tonight you have a standard meal. Caution —eat slowly, chew well, and don't let your appetite deceive you. Don't overeat! Your dinner should consist of a small portion of protein (meat, fish, poultry) one cooked vegetable (your choice) and a small amount of starch (bread, potatoes, rice, etc.). Go slow—eat intelligently. Too much will destroy everything you have been striving for.

000   Glasses Juice/Water Consumed
000000000   Glasses Water Consumed
0   Fruit Consumed
0   Salad Consumed
0   Standard Meal Consumed
000000   Energy Expenders Initiated
000   Additional Expenders?
000   Megatetic Tablets
000   Nutritional Supplements
0   Chart Updated

DAILY SCHEDULE

THURSDAY

DAY 28

2 Days to Final Goal   Starting Weight   Lbs.

Less Weight This AM   Lbs.

Equals Weight Loss   Lbs.

SUMMARY: You have gained again, probably! Don't be upset—it
was expected. As I have said before, the weight is no more important than the inches. Today eat as yesterday. Continue to expend
energy through additional tasks. Don't let down your guard—in
only two days you will have successfully completed your 30-day
program.

000   Glasses Juice/Water Consumed

000000000   Glasses Water Consumed

0   Fruit Consumed

0   Salad Consumed

0   Standard Meal Consumed

000000   Energy Expenders Initiated

000   Additional Expenders?

000   Megatetic Tablets

000   Nutritional Supplements

0   Chart Updated

DAILY SCHEDULE

FRIDAY

DAY 29

1 Day to Final Goal

Starting Weight	Lbs.
Less Weight This AM	Lbs.
Equals Weight Loss	Lbs.

SUMMARY: Slight loss of weight can be expected but is unnecessary. You should be feeling fine and should be right on schedule with your final goal tommorow. The dramatic changes that have taken place over the past month attest to your determination and strong will. After tomorrow you will be able to take pride in your accomplishment.

000   Glasses Juice/Water Consumed
000000000   Glasses Water Consumed
0   Fruit Consumed
0   Salad Consumed
0   Standard Meal Consumed
000000   Energy Expenders Initiated
000   Additional Expenders?
000   Megatetic Tablets
000   Nutritional Supplements
0   Chart Updated

DAILY SCHEDULE

SATURDAY

DAY 30

		Starting Weight	Lbs.
		Less Weight This AM	Lbs.
Final Goal	Lbs.	Equals Weight Loss	Lbs.

SUMMARY: It's over! Today you should be within one or two pounds of your final goal. Eat the same as yesterday. Tomorrow you will change to a standard dietary intake with only a few alterations. Congratulations! You deserve all those compliments you are receiving. You should reward yourself with new clothes or plans for a long-awaited vacation. New activities, increased energy and a slender body are all well deserved.

000 Glass Juice/Water Consumed
000000000 Glasses Water Consumed
0 Fruit Consumed
0 Salad Consumed
0 Standard Meal Consumed
000000 Energy Expenders Initiated
000 Additional Expenders?
000 Megatetic Tablets
000 Nutritional Supplements
0 Chart Updated

DAILY SCHEDULE

SUNDAY

DAY 31

SUMMARY: Today is your day of liberation. Use the suggestions in Chapter 9 and you will never again have to restrict your activities or be embarrassed about your weight. You have worked hard over the past thirty days to achieve your goals. In the future you will be able to control your weight without much effort—BUT—you will have to keep track of your progress. Chapters 9 and following contain everything you need to maintain your slenderness. Use the information in those chapters and you will never be fat again. Once again, congratulations!

CHARTING YOUR PROGRESS

As was said previously, keeping your weight loss on schedule is important. One method of visualizing your interim, as well as final goals, is to chart your progress. In this way you will be able to determine where you are and where you are going, at a glance. A few sample charts have been included in this chapter so that you can see the differences in weight loss patterns for various individuals. No one person can be said to be progressing properly through the program based solely on his chart. Yet, as you can see by these sample charts, each individual's progress falls within the boundaries of a broad corridor. If you follow the Megatetic Weight Reduction Program as directed, your chart should also fall within these boundaries.

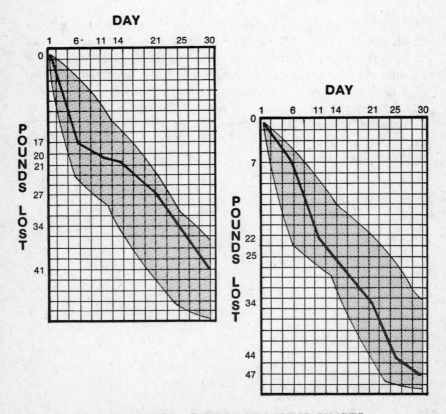

FIGURE 7-1: SAMPLE PROGRESS CHARTS

DAY

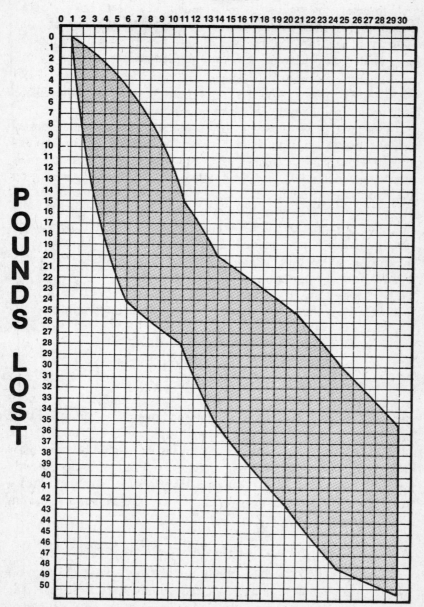

FIGURE 7-2: YOUR PROGRESS CHART

Keep your chart up-dated. By doing this, you will quickly be able to determine what steps must be taken to meet your next goal on schedule. There is no reason for you to be unaware of your progress at any time during your 30-day program. A quick look at your chart will determine how well you are doing.

Each day during your 30-day program you should record the number of pounds lost on the above chart. In this way you will be able to quickly determine your progress.

As long as your weight losses remain within the boundaries established, you are proceeding correctly and should not be concerned with small differences between your progress chart and your interim goals. Only if your chart reflects insufficient weight loss, by going outside the boundaries, should you re-evaluate your progress. See "Keeping Your Weight Loss on Schedule" on page 107.

For purposes of clarification only the weight on the interim goal days has been recorded. Note that although each pattern of weight loss differs dramatically, both progress charts reveal a successful program through sustained weight loss.

In both cases represented by these charts, the weight loss remained within the predetermined boundaries of the program.

USING THE ENVIRONMENT SCHEDULE TO BURN OFF THOSE EXTRA POUNDS

Most weight-reduction programs incorporate large numbers of routine exercises. These are usually boring, strenuous, and nonproductive. They can rarely be continued over long periods of time and therefore are usually dropped and forgotten in short order. The Megatetic Weight Reduction Program, as was stated previously, is based on the fact that most overweight people are that way not only because they are healthy, but also, extra efficient in their activities. I also believe that most overweight people hate monotonous, nonproductive exercises.

EXPENDING ENERGY WITHOUT EXERCISES

Fortunately, there is a way to use up extra calories; to burn off those extra pounds without standard or routine exercises. I call this method the "Energy Expender"; it was described in a previous chapter. Now, as you begin your 30-day weight-loss program it is time to use the Expender along with your Environment Schedule.

Most individuals perform the same basic tasks every day. Over the years this becomes routine, and each daily activity becomes less demanding, both physically and mentally. One way to increase your energy expenditure is to alter your daily tasks. Since you probably are very efficient in what you do, you must also change your environment sufficiently in an effort to expend more energy while performing the same basic tasks. This method works better than exercises because it can be continued for life and doesn't require any special time to be set aside. In addition, you don't have to "psych" yourself up as you might if you had to perform exercises.

Only once do you rearrange your environment and from that point on you will burn up hundreds and perhaps thousands of extra calories every day without giving it a second thought. Start by writing down your usual daily activities, trying to also include those things you do perhaps only once a week. Then go through this list and see how many things you can move or change which will help you burn off those extra pounds. Use your imagination; your creativity. It will be a whole new experience for you. Up until now you have done everything with a view to efficiency. It will take some thought to alter this. Study the following twelve suggestions. I am sure you will be able to come up with at least twelve more that will help you use up those unnecessary calories.

TWELVE WAYS TO USE UP CALORIES

1. Arise fifteen minutes earlier than at present. Even if you just want to lie in bed for those fifteen minutes, that's O.K. Lying awake burns up more calories than sleeping.
2. Move your alarm clock to the other side of the room. It will take several extra steps to shut it off. More calories burned!
3. Shower every day and if possible two or three times a day. You will feel better and at the same time rid yourself of those extra pounds.

4. For men: shave *every day*, even on those days off.

5. For women: wash your hair three or more times a week. Shampoo isn't essential if your hair is very fine. Cool water and a scalp massage will do nicely. It will also strengthen your hair.

6. Very few people brush their teeth more than once daily. Be sure to do this two or three times a day. Extra calories burned and stronger and healthier teeth will be the result.

7. Rearrange your kitchen cabinets. Put most-used items in out of the way places. Put dishes in under the counter cabinets. Separate utensils into two or three different drawers. Put cups and glasses farther away from sink, stove, or refrigerator. Putting the milk on a lower shelf will mean hundreds of extra calories burned annually.

8. Rearrange your medicine cabinet, or if you have more than one bathroom, try to use the one that will mean extra steps for you.

9. Rearrange closets and shelves. Choose the clothes closet furthest from where you normally get dressed.

10. If you take public transportation to work, get off one stop early. The walk of a few blocks will be excellent for you.

11. If you have an elevator at home or at business, walk up or down at least one flight each day.

12. When setting up work of any kind, reverse your normal procedure. Make the job just slightly more difficult or time consuming. In less than a week it will become second nature to you.

Don't forget! Change your environment on the third day of your Megatetic Weight Reduction Program and you won't have to worry about exercises. Add your own ideas to the above suggestions, as many as possible, it means thousands of extra calories.

8 | HOW TO LOSE TEN POUNDS IN ONE WEEK

10 days

$$7 da = 25$$
$$7 da = 5$$
$$7 da = 5$$
$$7 da = 5$$

40

```
12 10
  25
-----
 290
  25
-----
 185
```

```
 25
 15
---
 40
```

```
4 10
 40
----
170
```

```
2 10
 50
----
160
```

SAVINGS WITHDRAWAL

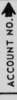

ACCOUNT NO. ⬆

DATE _____ 19 ___

PASSBOOK MUST BE PRESENTED WHEN FUNDS ARE WITHDRAWN

NORTHWEST NATIONAL BANK

RECEIVED FROM

DOLLARS $ _____

_____
SIGNATURE

_____
ADDRESS

TO BE CHARGED TO MY SAVINGS ACCOUNT

Teller's Initial
_____

DISPOSITION	
Cash	
Checking	

109 3/72

Some patients who successfully complete the 30-day Megatetic program return several months later seeking help. What often happens is that the newly slender patient becomes overconfident and fails to pay adequate attention to his dietary intake. In other cases, patients have put the blame on some special event such as a vacation trip, cruise, wedding, or other festive occasion. In any event, what has happened is that the once slender individual has regained several pounds. Many times they have tried to diet on their own only to find that, for them, the loss of five or ten pounds is extremely difficult.

In order to help these patients, a new program was developed. It is called the Mini-Megatetic program, and it is specifically formulated to assist the slightly overweight individual achieve a desirable weight level in one week or less.

IS THE MINI-MEGATETIC PROGRAM FOR YOU?

If you require weight loss in excess of ten pounds you should not use the Mini-Megatetic Program. It will only cause a prolongation of your overweight condition. For weight reduction in excess of ten pounds follow the full 30-day Megatetic Program. If you achieve your desirable weight prior to the 30-day period you have only to turn to Chapter 9 and proceed as directed. On the other hand, if ten pounds is the most you wish to lose the Mini-Megatetic Program will be just right for you. As in the 30-day program, if you achieve your desirable weight before completion of the program, turn to Chapter 9 and follow the instructions and re-orientation program as outlined.

HOW THE MINI-MEGATETIC PROGRAM WORKS

All too often the slightly overweight individual is led to believe that all that is necessary to lose a few pounds is a minimal reduction in food intake. This unfortunately is untrue! Slight reduction in consumption (unless continued for long periods of time) does little if anything to alter your weight. The reason for this is quite simple. In order for you to lose weight, you must consume less food than is necessary to *maintain* your present weight. In other words, your intake of food must be *less* than your energy expenditure. Since the act of eating, digesting and metabolizing food uses up calories, the benefits which might accrue from a slight decrease in food intake is partially offset by reduced energy expenditure. This decreased energy expenditure is the result of not having to digest and metabolize the small additional amount of food you had been eating. Therefore, in order for you to lose any significant amount of weight you would have to strictly adhere to a dietary program of this nature for several weeks, and perhaps even months.

To overcome the disadvantages of such a prolonged and tedious approach to the loss of a few pounds, the Mini-Megatetic Program was designed. By reducing normal food intake dramatically (for a short period of time) the Mini-Megatetic Program produces rapid weight loss and assists you in formulating new dietary habits through the following re-orientation program presented in Chapter 9.

Follow the program, as outlined, for a *maximum* of seven days and you will be amazed at the number of pounds you lose.

HOW TO LOSE THOSE FEW EXTRA POUNDS FAST

In order to achieve your goals, follow *all* the recommendations and advice in the same way you would if you were going to utilize the full 30-day program. Don't be misled into thinking that since you only have a few pounds to lose you won't need to chart your progress or follow directions exactly. The only difference in the Mini-Megatetic Program as compared to the full 30-day program is that it is designed to produce a more easily followed regimen over a shorter period of time. This is possible only because the total number of pounds to be lost is minimal.

Once again, proceed in the same manner as for the full 30-day program with the following modification: *Instead of using the 30 Daily Schedules as presented in Chapter 7, substitute the following Seven Daily Schedules.* In one week or less you will have achieved your goals.

DAILY SCHEDULE

FRIDAY

DAY 1

SUMMARY: Today will be your first day of fasting. And today you will consume nothing but water. Upon arising check your weight, as this will be your starting weight for the purposes of your seven day program. Since dinner last evening you should not have taken any food or drink. You will be able to get through this first day with little difficulty. Around lunch time you may feel tired or perhaps "jittery". This is to be expected and should be ignored. You may also note some stomach "growling" as your digestive tract reacts to the absence of food. This too will pass shortly and should not give you any concern.

If you should find this first day's fast too difficult it is permissable to drink one 4 ounce glass of fruit juice (of your choice) mixed with 4 ounces of water. Sip this mixture to alleviate the "jitteriness" or "growling" stomach. If you can do without the juice/water mixture, however, so much the better. You will probably find that you are more tired than usual this evening. This is normal and is the result of lowered blood sugar. Get plenty of rest this evening.

Fill in the following information on your calendar:

Starting Weight	Lbs.
Less Desired Weight	Lbs.
Equals Final Weight	
Loss Goal	Lbs.

And prepare this Checklist:
    Starting Weight Determined
    Final Goal Determined
    Nutritional Supplement Upon Arising
    Visual Goals Clipped and Placed
    Chart Started (page 140, Chapter 7)
    9 Glasses of Water Consumed
    1 Glass of Juice/Water Mixture Consumed?

2 Days to Interim Goal

DAILY SCHEDULE

SATURDAY

DAY 2

SUMMARY: This morning you may feel as if you didn't get enough sleep last night. This is not unusual and will slowly pass as the day moves on. Nothing to eat or drink today except water. You may be bothered by a headache, and if this does occur, lie down and rest in a darkened room. Drink extra water, and the headache will soon pass as the increased toxins in your bloodstream are eliminated. No juice/water mixture intake today. You should still have bowel movements although they may be diminishing.

Fill in the following information on your calendar:

    Starting Weight   Lbs.
    Less Weight This AM   Lbs.
    Equals Weight Loss   Lbs.

And prepare this Checklist:

    List of Daily Activities (page 141, Chapter 7)
    9 Glasses of Water Consumed
    Chart Updated
    7 Ways to Increase Energy Expenditure
1 Day to Interim Goal

DAILY SCHEDULE

SUNDAY

DAY 3

SUMMARY: This morning you should reach your first interim goal. Tomorrow you will once again begin to take food. Do not allow yourself to slip backwards. This morning you may notice a coating on your tongue and a disagreeable breath odor. This is indicative of continued toxin removal from your system. It is normal, and shouldn't concern you. You may feel tired most of the day. Rest often for short periods of time if this should occur.

You should already notice a loss of puffiness, and clothes that were "snug" last week should fit comfortably by this afternoon.

Fill in the following information on your calendar:

Starting Weight	Lbs.
Less Weight This AM	Lbs.
Equals Weight Loss	Lbs.

And prepare this Checklist:
    9 Glasses of Water Consumed
    Changed Environment in Preparation of Energy Expender
    Chart Updated

Interim Goal 4 Lbs. Lost

DAILY SCHEDULE

MONDAY

DAY 4

SUMMARY: Today begins the second phase of your program. You may have one glass of the juice/water mixture as well as one piece of fruit. An apple is recommended.

You need not drink the full glass of the mixture or eat the entire apple at one time—it would be better if you took small sips of the juice and one slice of the apple several times throughout the day. Diarrhea may be present, but is generally of short duration. Continue to drink adequate amounts of water.

Fill in the following information on your calendar:

Starting Weight	Lbs.
Less Weight This AM	Lbs.
Equals Weight Loss	Lbs.

And prepare this Checklist:
9 Glasses of Water Consumed
Energy Expender Initiated
Chart Updated
1 Glass Juice/Water Mixture Consumed
1 Nutritional Supplement Taken with Juice/Water Mixture
1 Piece of Fruit Consumed
1 Megatetic Tablet Taken Prior to Solid Food

3 Days to Final Goal

DAILY SCHEDULE

TUESDAY

DAY 5

SUMMARY: This morning you may notice a slight gain of weight. This is to be expected. Your body is beginning to retain small amounts of the fluids you are taking in. Don't be concerned about this. Today you will drink and eat the same as yesterday. Diarrhea should pass and your tongue should resume its normal pinkish tone if it hasn't already done so. Tomorrow begins the third and final phase of your program. Don't let anyone divert you from your goals.

Fill in the following information on your calendar:

Starting Weight	Lbs.
Less Weight This AM	Lbs.
Equals Weight Loss	Lbs.

And prepare this Checklist:

9 Glasses of Water Consumed
1 Glass of Juice/Water Mixture Consumed
1 Nutritional Supplement Taken with Juice/Water Mixture
1 Piece of Fruit Consumed
1 Megatetic Tablet Taken Prior to Solid Food
Chart Updated
Energy Expenders Utilized

2 Days to Final Goal

DAILY SCHEDULE

WEDNESDAY

DAY 6

SUMMARY: Tomorrow is your final day of the program. Do not allow yourself to become sidetracked. You should notice a slight loss of weight this morning. Today you may consume two glasses of the Juice/Water Mixture, but do not eat any solid fruit. With only tomorrow left I know you want to achieve your final goal on schedule. You may notice some craving for food today. Disregard it—tomorrow is your last day on the program. By now you should be noticing a marked reduction in your size. Your clothing should be quite loose-fitting.

Fill in the following information on your calendar:

Starting Weight	Lbs.
Less Weight This AM	Lbs.
Equals Weight Loss	Lbs.

And prepare this Checklist:
- 9 Glasses of Water Consumed
- 2 Glasses of Juice/Water Mixture Consumed
- 2 Nutritional Supplements Taken with Juice/Water Mixture
- Energy Expenders Utilized
- Chart Updated

1 Day to Final Goal

DAILY SCHEDULE

THURSDAY

DAY 7

SUMMARY: Today is your last day on the program. You should have achieved, or possibly surpassed your desired weight loss. If you still have a short way to go you will most likely lose those last remaining pounds by morning. Do not alter your intake today. Two glasses of Juice/Water Mixture is all that is allowed. Tomorrow you will be eating again so don't throw everything you've achieved away be overindulging today.

Congratulations on your rapid weight loss!

Tomorrow you should begin to follow the re-orientation program as presented in Chapter 9.

Fill in the following information on your calendar:

Starting Weight	Lbs.
Less Weight This AM	Lbs.
Equals Weight Loss	Lbs.

And prepare this Checklist:

9 Glasses of Water Consumed

2 Glasses of Juice/Water Mixture Consumed

2 Nutritional Supplements Taken with Juice/Water Mixture

Energy Expenders Utilized

Chart Updated

Final Goal 10 Lbs.

9 | ADJUSTING TO A SLENDER WAY OF LIFE

You've achieved your ultimate goal and now you're slender! Your body feels great and I'm sure that today is one of the happiest days of your life. It was difficult, but now it's over. For the rest of your life you will be proud of your figure. You will no longer have to be defensive. You will be able to take part in all those activities you enjoy and never again be embarassed by your obesity.

Friends and relatives are remarking about how good you look, and I am sure that you never again want to be fat.

If you will follow the directions and recommendations contained in this and succeeding chapters, you will never have to fear overweight again. Do not become complacent! You have worked hard to achieve your slenderness. Do not allow complacency to rob you of your success. The Megatetic Program contains everything you need to maintain life-long slenderness. Use it and you will always be proud of your figure, always happy with your slenderness.

HOW TO ENJOY REORIENTATION

Getting back to a normal routine is sometimes difficult. The abrupt change which occurs when one is no longer "on a diet" can be very distressing. Psychologists have found that rapid changes in lifestyle produce enormous psychological and emotional stresses. It is for this reason that astronauts are given an extended period of de-briefing and reorientation when they return from a mission. Individuals about to be discharged from military service, returning prisoners of war, and even businessmen at the mercy of jet-lag, require at least a short transition period before becoming involved in routine activities. In this same way, dieters who are no longer on a strict, regimented program, need a short period of re-adjustment. To complete a dietary program one day and try to return to a normal routine the next, is foolhardy. The emotional stresses are too great and temptation is everywhere. Since you have been so successful, I am sure you don't want to regain those unsightly pounds. It is for this reason that the following reorientation program was formulated. It will make those first days after the program enjoyable. By following the procedure exactly as outlined you will have no trouble readjusting to a normal everyday routine. You will be eating properly. Both the quantity and quality of food has been taken into consideration and you should not alter them in any way. Do not allow others to coax you into having "just a little more" or "just try a little of this." They have not worked as you have to achieve slenderness—don't let their well-meaning, but misplaced concern rob you of all you've achieved.

YOUR ONE WEEK REORIENTATION PROGRAM

The material contained in the following pages has been designed to make transition from your 30-day program to normal eating habits, as easy, safe, and enjoyable as possible.

The combinations and quantities of food are inter-related and therefore substitutions are not recommended. Eat slowly, chew your food well, and never . . . *never* skip a meal.

By the end of one week your body will have readjusted to a normal dietary intake. At that time you should be both physically and psychologically ready to determine what and how much food you shoud eat in the future.

During your one week reorientation you may notice either a gain or loss of several pounds. This is to be expected and is of no consequence. Although you should continue to weigh yourself daily (keeping records) the alteration which may occur in your weight during the reorientation program will be minimal. Once you return to a normal eating pattern your weight will become stabilized and at that time care must be taken not to overlook the gain or loss of a pound or two.

REORIENTATION PROGRAM
DAY 1
Breakfast

1 multi-vitamin

4 oz. orange juice

½ cup dry fortified cereal (i.e., Rice Crispies, Cheerios, corn flakes) may be sweetened with sugar substitute

4 oz. whole milk

Tea or coffee as desired (black or use part of milk allowance, no sugar—sugar substitute may be used)

Lunch

2 slices processed cheese

2 saltine crackers *or* 2 melba toast

4 oz. grapefruit juice mixed with 4 oz. of water

Tea or coffee as above

Dinner

1 pork chop or lamb chop, broiled (½ to ¾″ thick)

½ cup cooked green beans

2 tbs. mashed potatoes (made with water)

1 pat butter

Tea or coffee as above

REORIENTATION PROGRAM
DAY 2
Breakfast

1 multi-vitamin
4 oz. orange juice
½ cup dry fortified cereal (i.e., Rice Crispies, Cheerios, corn flakes) may be sweetened with sugar substitute
4 oz. whole milk
Tea or coffee as desired (black—or use part of milk allowance, no sugar—sugar substitute may be used)

Lunch

1 poached egg
1 sl. dry toast (rye or whole wheat)
4 oz. of juice of your choice mixed with 4 oz. water
Tea or coffee as above

Dinner

2 sl. (each approx. ¼″ thick by 3″ dia.) roasted meat, fish or fowl
1 cup loosely packed lettuce and tomato salad (may be seasoned with 1 tbs. salad oil and vinegar and spices to taste)
Tea and coffee as above

REORIENTATION PROGRAM

DAY 3

Breakfast

1 multi-vitamin
4 oz. unsweetened prune juice
½ cup cooked cereal (i.e., oatmeal, farina, Wheatena) may be
   sweetened with sugar substitute
4 oz. whole milk

Tea or coffee as desired (black—or use part of milk allowance, no
   sugar—sugar substitute may be used)

Lunch

2 sl. tomato on lettuce leaf
4 oz. creamed cottage cheese
2 saltine crackers *or* 2 melba toast

Tea or coffee as above

Dinner

1 chicken leg and thigh (broiled or roasted)
½ cup cooked rice
½ pat butter
1 small apple

Tea or coffee as above

REORIENTATION PROGRAM
DAY 4
Breakfast

1 multi-vitamin

4 oz. unsweetened prune juice

½ cup cooked cereal (i.e., oatmeat, farina, Wheatena) may be sweetened with sugar substitute

4 oz. whole milk

Tea or coffee as desired (black—or use part of milk allowance, no sugar—sugar substitute may be used)

Lunch

2 sl. luncheon meat of your choice

1 cup loosely packed lettuce and tomato salad (may be seasoned with 1 tbs salad oil and vinegar and spices to taste)

1 sl. bread (rye or whole wheat)

Tea or coffee as above

Dinner

4 oz. whole milk

1 filet of flounder or other fish (broiled or poached)

½ cup cooked chopped broccoli

2 tbs. mashed potatoes (made with water)

½ banana

Tea or coffee as above

REORIENTATION PROGRAM
DAY 5
Breakfast

1 multi-vitamin
4 oz. orange juice
½ cup dry fortified cereal (i.e., Rice Crispies, Cheerios, corn flakes) may be sweetened with sugar substitute
4 oz. whole milk

Tea or coffee as desired (black—or use part of milk allowance, no sugar—sugar substitute may be used)

Lunch

2 sl. luncheon meat of your choice
½ cup cooked green beans
1 sl. bread (rye or whole wheat)
1 small apple

Tea or coffee as above

Dinner

4 oz. whole milk
1 pork chop or lamb chop, broiled (½ to ¾" thick)
½ cup cooked mixed vegetables
½ cup cooked rice
1 pat butter
½ pear in own juices

Tea or coffee as above

REORIENTATION PROGRAM
DAY 6
Breakfast

1 multi-vitamin
4 oz. unsweetened prune juice
1 poached egg
1 sl. dry toast (rye or whole wheat)

Tea or coffee as desired (black—or use part of milk allowance, no
   sugar—sugar substitute may be used)

Lunch

4 oz. whole milk
2 sl. tomato on lettuce leaf
2 sl. luncheon meat of your choice
1 sl. bread
1 small apple

Tea or coffee as above

Dinner

4 oz. whole milk
1 hamburger pattie, broiled (approx. 4 oz.)
½ cup cooked lima beans
1 sl. bread
½ cup fruit salad in own juices

Tea or coffee as above

REORIENTATION PROGRAM

DAY 7

Breakfast

1 multi-vitamin
4 oz. tomato juice
1 poached egg
1 sl. dry toast

Tea or coffee as desired (black—or use part of milk allowance, no
   sugar—sugar substitute may be used)

Lunch

1 hamburger pattie, broiled (approx. 4 oz.)
½ cup creamed cottage cheese
2 sl. tomato on lettuce leaf
1 small apple

Tea or coffee as above

Dinner

4 oz. whole milk
1 sl. roasted meat, fish or fowl (approx. ¾″ × 3″)
½ cup corn niblets
½ cup mashed potatoes (made with water)
1 pat butter
½ banana if desired

Tea or coffee as above

10 THE WONDERFUL WORLD OF SLENDERNESS

Being slender is an entirely new experience for you, and it will undoubtedly take some time to get used to it. Since you have already completed your seven day re-orientation, you will now be starting on the Megatetic Post-Program Procedure. By following this procedure, as outlined in Chapters 10 and 11, you will never have to worry about obesity again.

At the same time, however, you must learn to live with your new slenderness. You have been overweight for a long time, and although your body is now slender, your mental image of yourself will take some time to change. You have thought of yourself as fat for so long that slenderness is a difficult concept to comprehend (on a sub-conscious level).

In order to make slenderness a permanent part of your life you will not only require a slender body but also, you will have to think and act slender. The following recommendations will help you do just that.

HOW TO REMOVE OBSTACLES TO
PERMANENT SLENDERNESS

Now that you have lost all that excess weight, the clothing you were wearing no longer fits properly. Even clothes that you bought during the 30-day program probably look awkward on you. Your first priority therefore, is to obtain a new wardrobe. If you cannot afford a complete new set of clothes, at least purchase the basics as required by your lifestyle. There is nothing more pathetic than seeing a slender person swishing around in clothes that are several sizes too large. I make this recommendation from past experience. I have watched many patients who refused to get rid of their oversized clothing, slowly and gradually start to fill them again. Get rid of your old clothes. Destroy them or give them away; but be sure to get them out of your house.

A second major requirement of thinking slender is to drop your defenses. All the time you were overweight you were undoubtedly defensive, using various rationales, ploys, and excuses to protect your ego. This is natural and is seen in almost every overweight person. Now that you are no longer fat, you no longer need to be defensive. You will have to consciously work at this since your defensive nature is deeply imbedded. I have personally found that most overweight individuals respond to quips about their weight in a generous and good-natured way. At the same time, however, criticism about any thing other than their weight, meets with immediate and ruthless responses. This is known as psychological substitution, and is one way the obese individual protects his ego. It is considered socially rude for an obese person to take offense at remarks about his weight (yet ironically, it is not considered bad taste for a slender person to make such remarks). Therefore, he usually overlooks any references made in that area and substitutes another activity area which he protects with vehemence. If you will think back over the events of the past six months, you will probably be able to recall an instance that correlates with what I have been saying. You will probably be able to remember a time when you over-reacted in an extreme and possibly irrational manner to a seemingly harmless remark about this or that.

Since obesity is no longer an area of contention, you must neutralize your defensive behavior regarding your particular substitution activity area. In this way you will be able to normalize your response and look upon obesity as you truly feel about it subconsciously. This psychological alteration will help you remain slender in the future. Your true feelings about being fat will partially prevent you form overeating and therefore prevent you regaining weight.

Once you accomplish these two major objectives:
1) Wearing clothing which fits properly
2) Removing or neutralizing your defensive behavior regarding obesity,

you will be ready to truly "Think Slender."

HOW LURLENE McC. CHANGED HER PSYCHOLOGICAL OUTLOOK

Lurlene McC. had been grossly overweight ever since the birth of her first child some 14 years previously. When she first entered the office, she was 38 years old, a mother of two and a devoted wife. Her weight at that time was 168 pounds. Lurlene reported that she had been successful in losing weight on several previous occasions, but always managed to regain.

During her 30-day program Lurlene lost 43 pounds; an excellent reduction. I spent many hours with Lurlene during her program and explained in detail the mechanism of psychological substitution. Today, more than 18 months after her initial program, Lurlene is still maintaining her desirable weight On a recent visit to the office, I asked her what she thought was primarily responsible for her continued slenderness. Lurlene McC. related the following story:

"Although every part of the post-program procedure has given me some help in maintaining my weight, I think the major thing for me was the change in my psychological outlook.

"I had never realized it before, but when I was overweight, I used to make jokes about being fat. I was the proverbial 'jolly fat person.' When others used to kid me about it, I used to laugh it off. It wasn't until you explained psychological substitution to me that I realized how defensive I was about my family and especially my husband. Apparently I had substituted protection of my family for protection of my ego. I am sure that most women are defensive when it comes to criticism about their families, but my reactions to comments concerning my husband or children were definitely out of balance.

"I remember one occasion in particular when Doris R., a close friend and neighbor, remarked that Tom (Lurlene's husband) didn't seem to do much work around the house. My reaction to that seemingly innocuous statement was to almost physically throw her out of my house. I verbally destroyed her. I ranted and raved, and criticized Doris in terms which I would now be ashamed to repeat.

"I didn't realize it at the time but my reactions were definitely based on a fear of losing my husband to another woman. Deep down inside I knew that my fatness was displeasing to Tom and so I tried in other ways to make him happy around the house. I never asked him to do anything. Any repairs that had to be done, I did.

"Now that I am slender, I no longer react as violently as before. I realize that fear was the motivating factor and I have been very fortunate in being able to work out my anxieties. I still love my husband and children as much as ever, but I no longer feel threatened when someone makes a remark about them.

"I think now I am asserting myself properly. I take a dim view of remarks about my previous obesity—I no longer wish to discuss it or make fun of it. I take it seriously and refuse to allow it to become the butt of jokes. I think I've done a good job rearranging my concerns about my family and my obesity. I don't think I'll ever be fat again."

HOW TO ENJOY THINKING SLENDER

Now that you have made a commitment to dress and behave as a slender person would, it is important for you to train yourself to think in the same way. You may be shocked to learn that during the time you were overweight you were thinking "fat", yet this is true nonetheless.

Instead of reinforcing this kind of thinking by explaining it in detail, I will present the other side of the coin and demonstrate what is meant by thinking "thin". Very simply stated, thinking "thin" requires only that you ask yourself the following question before performing any act:

"What would a thin (slender) person do?"

If you do nothing more than ask this question, and then proceed to act in accordance with the answer, you will never again be overweight. You need not concern yourself with the related questions of why, where, when, who and how, as these will remain constant.

Why?—Because I want to remain slender.
Where?—Here.
When?—Now.
Who?—Slender me.
How?—As a slender person would.

Therfore, all you must determine is *what* a slender person would do when faced with any particular set of circumstances. By doing this, thinking slender will not only be an effective deterrent to obesity but it will also become an enjoyable approach to action.

ACTING SLENDER OFFERS TWO BENEFITS

As you begin asking yourself, "What would a slender person do?" you will begin to act as a slender person would. This will result in at least two major benefits. First, you will be able to enjoy all the activities that slender people enjoy and second, you will be able to maintain your new lowered weight.

WHY GENE D. HASN'T REGAINED ANY WEIGHT

Gene had been overweight ever since he could remember. Now at age 34 he had finally reduced his weight and was determined to keep it down.

In order to prevent his regaining, Gene formulated the following statement, and repeats it to himself at least a dozen times a day:

I'll never let another do,
What I can do as well.
I'll never eat without much thought
And thereby always feel swell.

Gene told me that many times each day he finds himself in a position where he could easily forget himself and begin to regain pounds. By repeating the above statement at such times, he feels that he has prevented himself from becoming lazy or eating improperly.

"Because of my job," Gene told me, "I often find myself in a position where I can either do something myself or have one of my subordinates do it.

"By following the requirements of my statement, I find that I accomplish as much as ever and at the same time use up extra calories. When I find myself in a restaurant or sitting down to eat, the second part of my statement prevents me from overdoing it. I think everyone who wants to remain slender should make up a simple statement that will serve as a reminder to do more and eat less."

THE FUTURE: SLENDERNESS FOREVER

You are now just about ready to proceed on your own. Before you do, however, you should make a commitment to perpetual slenderness. It won't be the easiest thing for you to do, but if you apply yourself, and make use of the recommendations found in this and succeeding chapters, you will soon find that slenderness can be habit forming.

From time to time you may be indiscreet in choosing what and how much you eat. But by paying attention to how you feel and how much you weigh, you will soon be able to control your weight within very strict limits. All in all, if you continue with your Energy Expender program, you will have little to worry about.

Be sure to keep an eye on your weight though. A gain of one or two pounds is of little consequence, but anything over that indicates a return to obesity. If you find yourself putting on a few pounds, take immediate steps to reverse the process. The additional suggestions contained in Chapter 12 will be invaluable in this regard. By all means, though, pay attention to your weight. Do not disregard even slight changes in your daily activities or eating habits. By doing this you will remain slender forever.

HOW TO MAINTAIN YOUR WEIGHT WITH THE ENERGY EXPENDER

If, during your 30-day program you properly followed instructions, you will, by now, have initiated several energy expenders. These, of course, helped you lose those excess pounds fast. Now, if you will conitnue to incorporate increased energy expenditure into your lifestyle, you will continue to use up those extra calories. Small indiscretions will not affect your stabilized weight. You will be able to indulge yourself on those special occasions, without fear of ever being fat again. The Energy Expender program will remain, for the rest of your life, as a guardian against obesity. Use it to its full potential. Approach your future in an intelligent and logical manner, and you will never have to be concerned about obesity again.

SCHEDULING IS ALL IMPORTANT

As you now move on, you'll have a tendency to forget yourself from time to time. You may eat too much or perhaps do too little. For this reason you should schedule your use of the Energy Expender system appropriately. Pick one day each week—the same day, and note on your calendar, "EE." In this way you will remind yourself that you should think about energy expenditure on that day. Be sure that you do not disregard the note nor postpone consideration of what must be done.

Each week when that particular day arrives, set some time aside to formulate a new energy expender unit. This may require some time and effort on your part, but it will be more than worth it in the long run. Don't be discouraged—resolve that you will not proceed with other chores until you have devised at least one additional energy expender.

Once you do decide on one—initiate the change immediately. Rearrange whatever fixtures or furnishings must be moved. If your idea means doing more, begin at once—don't procrastinate. Initiate your program and follow through. In just a week or two your energy expender will become second nature to you. You will continue with it and your other expenders for life, and thus will continue to maintain your weight through holidays, special occasions, and all those other times which may have, in the past, caused a regain of weight.

II THE EASY WAY TO EVERLASTING SLENDERNESS

Since the Megatetic Program is designed not only to produce rapid weight loss, but also to permanently maintain your slenderness, it is now time for you to decide on the long-range method of staying slim which is best suited for you.

Each individual has different needs and desires, and therefore any long-range program must be designed specifically for them. In the following pages I will present three basic approaches to maintaining slenderness along with two additional ways of removing excess pounds before they become permanent. You may decide to follow one or another, or you may intermingle the various approaches as desired so as to produce a long-range program which works for you. For instance—during the week you may decide that one approach works nicely, while on weekends or when going out to dinner, another approach is more suitable. By setting up your program accordingly, you will be able to enjoy yourself without gaining weight.

After reading over each of the three approaches, decide for yourself which method or combination best suits your needs. Try to set up a routine so as to make any conscious effort of following your program minimal. But don't hesitate to "mix and match" as you feel necessary. Each of the three methods is described on a daily basis so as to provide you with the greatest flexibility possible.

METHOD #1: THREE BALANCED MEALS A DAY

Many individuals find that their lifestyle and most of their daily activities are routine and repetitive. Certain periods of time are designated for work, others for relaxation, eating, or other activities. When this is the case, eating three meals a day is usually (but not always) best. Since the day is divided, and three meal times are designated, it is often best to use these times as intended.

To use this approach to maintaining your desirable weight level find your present desired weight on Chart A (Women) or Chart B (Men).

CHART A: WEIGHT MAINTENANCE FOR WOMEN

Desired Weight to be Maintained	Approx. Calories Permitted	Number of Servings to be Eaten Daily						
		Meat	Vegetable	Fruit	Milk	Bread	Fat	Sugar
101-110	1260	4.5	4.5	3.0	1.0	5.0	3.0	3.0
111-120	1380	5.0	5.5	3.0	1.5	6.0	3.0	3.0
121-130	1500	5.5	6.0	4.0	1.5	6.0	3.0	3.0 *2 sugars*
131-140	1620	6.0	7.0	4.0	2.0	7.0	3.0	3.0
141-150	1740	6.0	8.0	4.5	2.0	7.0	3.0	3.0
151-160	1860	6.5	8.5	5.0	2.0	8.0	3.0	3.0
161-170	1980	7.0	9.5	5.5	2.0	8.0	3.0	3.0
171-180	2100	7.5	10.0	6.0	2.0	9.0	3.0	3.0

Note: If your desired weight ends in a 1, 2 or 3 (i.e., 121, 122 or 123) eliminate one sugar and one fat from your daily intake. If your desired weight ends in a 4, 5 or 6 (i.e., 124, 125 or 126) eliminate one sugar from your daily intake. If your desired weight ends in a 7, 8, 9 or 0 (i.e., 127, 128, 129 or 130) follow the chart recommendations.

CHART B: WEIGHT MAINTENANCE FOR MEN

Desired Weight to be Maintained	Approx. Calories Permitted	Meat	Vegetable	Fruit	Milk	Bread	Fat	Sugar
111-120	1725	6.0	8.0	4.5	2.0	5.0	3.0	3.0
121-130	1875	6.5	9.0	5.0	2.0	5.5	3.0	3.0
131-140	2025	7.0	10.0	5.5	2.0	6.0	3.0	3.0
141-150	2175	7.5	11.0	6.0	2.5	6.0	3.0	3.0
151-160	2325	8.0	12.0	6.5	2.5	6.5	3.0	3.0
161-170	2475	9.0	13.0	7.0	2.5	7.0	3.0	3.0
171-180	2625	9.0	14.0	8.0	3.0	7.5	3.0	3.0
181-190	2775	10.0	15.0	8.5	3.0	8.0	3.0	3.0
191-200	2925	10.5	16.0	9.0	3.0	8.0	3.0	3.0
201-210	3075	11.0	17.0	9.5	3.0	8.5	3.0	3.0
211-220	3225	11.5	18.0	10.0	3.5	9.0	3.0	3.0
221-230	3375	12.0	19.0	10.5	3.5	9.5	3.0	3.0

The heading "Number of Servings to be Eaten Daily" spans the columns Meat, Vegetable, Fruit, Milk, Bread, Fat, Sugar.

Note: If your desired weight ends in a 1, 2 or 3 (i.e., 121, 122 or 123) eliminate one sugar and one fat from your daily intake. If your desired weight ends in a 4, 5 or 6 (i.e., 124, 125 or 126) eliminate one sugar from your daily intake. If your desired weight ends in a 7, 8, 9 or 0 (i.e., 127, 128, 129 or 130) follow the chart recommendations.

By reading across the chart you will then find the number of servings of different foods you are permitted to eat in any one 24-hour period. Noting the number of servings permitted, turn to the Food Category List on Page 184 and formulate your own daily menus according to your particular desires.

The following sample menu (for a woman who wishes to maintain a weight of 113 pounds) has been prepared as an example of how to use the Food Category List. (See page 185.)

SAMPLE DAILY INTAKE

Woman, 113 pound desirable weight:

By looking at Chart A you will find that a woman of this weight should eat the following kinds and amounts of food each day:

Meat	5.0 servings
Vegetables	5.5 servings
Fruit	3.0 servings
Milk	1.5 servings
Bread	6.0 servings
Fats	2.0 servings
Sugar	2.0 servings

Note: Since the desired weight ends in a 3, one fat and one sugar has been eliminated from the daily intake.

FOOD CATEGORY LIST

The following items may be used as desired and need not be measured:

Seasonings: Cinnamon, celery salt, garlic, garlic salt, lemon, mustard, mint, nutmeg, parsley, pepper, saccharine, and other sugarless sweeteners, all spices, vanilla, vinegar.

Raw Vegetables: Raw vegetables and their juices may be taken as desired. You should, however, indicate 0.5 servings (no matter how much you eat) under the vegetable category each time you eat raw vegetables.

Cabbage	Lettuce
Carrots	Peppers (red or green)
Celery	Stringbeans
Chicory	Tomatoes
Cucumbers	Watercress
Escarole	

SAMPLE DAILY MENU

—113 pound woman—

	Meat	Veg.	Fruit	Milk	Bread	Fat	Sugar
Breakfast:							
½ cup vegetable juice		0.5					
2 eggs, poached	2						
2 sl. toast, lightly buttered (1 tsp)					2	1	
2 tsp grape jam							2
Coffee, as desired with whole milk, and non-caloric sweetener (may be taken throughout the day)				0.5			
Lunch:							
1 broiled hamburger	1				2		
on a hamburger bun							
1 cup lettuce & tomato salad with		0.5					
1 tsp salad oil & vinegar to taste						1	
1 8 oz glass whole milk				1			
1 small apple			1				
Snack:							
1 raw carrot, 2 stalks celery		0.5					
Dinner							
½ grapefruit			1				
2 lamb chops	2						
1 cup carrots		2					
1 cup stringbeans		2					
2 small potatoes					2		
½ cup applesauce			1				
TOTALS	5.0	5.5	3.0	1.5	6.0	2.0	2.0

Other Foods: Coffee or tea (you may use a part or all of your milk and sugar allowances in the coffee or tea if desired), fat-free broth, bouillon, sour or dill pickles, cranberries, rhubarb.

The following foods should be eaten in accordance with the recommendations found in Chart A or B.

Meat Category:

Meat & Poultry (beef, lamb, pork, liver, chicken, etc.)	1 slice (3″ × 2″ × ¼″)
Cold Cuts (luncheon meats)	1 slice (4½″ square × ¼″
Frankurter	1 (8 to 9 per pound)
Codfish, Mackerel, etc.	1 slice (2″ × 2″ × 1″)
Salmon, Tuna, Crab	¼ cup
Oyster, Shrimp, Clams	5 small
Sardines	3 medium
Cheese, American, Swiss, Cheddar	1 slice (3″ × 2″ × ¼″)
Cheese, Cottage	¼ cup
Egg	1
Peanut Butter	2 tablespoons

Vegetable Category: COOKED - ½ Cup of Each Per Serving

Asparagus	Lettuce
Beets	Mushrooms
Broccoli	Okra
Brussel Sprouts	Onions
Cabbage	Peas, Green
Cauliflower	Peppers (red or green)
Carrots	Pumpkin
Celery	Rutabagas
Chicory	Sauerkraut
Cucumbers	Stringbeans
Eggplant	Squash, winter or summer
Escarole	Tomatoes

Greens: beet, chard	Turnip
collard, dandelion,	Watercress
kale, mustard	
spinach, turnip	

Fruit Category: May be fresh, dried, canned or frozen without sugar.

Apple	1 small (2″ dia.)
Applesauce	½ cup
Apricots, fresh	2 medium
Apricots, dried	4 halves
Banana	½ of small
Berries	1 cup
Blueberries	⅔ cup
Cantaloupe	¼ (6″ dia.)
Cherries	10 large
Dates	2
Figs, fresh	2 large
Figs, dried	1 small
Grapefruit	½ small
Grapefruit juice	½ cup
Grapes	12
Grapejuice	¼ cup
Honeydew Melon	⅛ (7″ dia.)
Mango	½ small
Orange	1 small
Orange Juice	½ cup
Papaya	⅓ medium
Peach	1 medium
Pear	1 small
Pineapple	½ cup
Pineapple juice	⅓ cup
Plums	2 medium
Prunes	2
Raisins	2 tablespoons
Tangerine	1 large
Watermelon	1 cup

Milk Category:

| Milk, whole | 1 cup |

Milk, evaporated	½ cup
Milk, skim or powered	1 cup + 2 fat allowances
Buttermilk	1 cup
Ice Cream	½ cup
Ice Milk	½ cup + 2 fat allowances
Light Cream	5 tablespoons
Heavy Cream	3 tablespoons

Bread Category:

Beans, baked (no pork)	¼ cup
Beans, lima, navy, etc.	½ cup
Bread	1 slice
Bread, low carbohydrate	1 slice
Biscuit	1 (2″ dia.)
Cereal, cooked	½ cup
Cereal, dry (flake or puffed)	¾ cup
Corn	⅓ cup
Cornbread	1½″ cube
Crackers: Graham	2
Oyster	20 (½ cup)
Round	6 to 8
Saltine	5
Soda	3
Flour	2 ½ tablespoons
Muffin	1 (2″ dia.)
Peas, split	½ cup
Potato, white, baked or boiled	1 (2″ dia.)
Potato, white, mashed	½ cup
Potato, sweet or yam	¼ cup
Rice or grits, cooked	½ cup
Roll	1 (2″ dia.)
Spaghetti, noodles, etc., cooked	½ cup
Sponge Cake	1 ½″ cube

Fat Category:

Butter or Margarine	1 teaspoon

Bacon, crisp	1 slice
Cream Cheese	1 tablespoon
French Dressing	1 tablespoon
Mayonnaise	1 teaspoon
Oil or Cooking Fat	1 teaspoon
Nuts	6 small
Olives	5 small
Avocado	⅛ (4″ dia.)

Sugar Category:

Beverages, carbonated: all, including cola type	4 oz.
Gelatin Dessert	½ cup
Honey	½ tablespoon
Jams, marmalades, preserves, jellies	1 tablespoon
Molasses	1 tablespoon
Pretzels	10 small sticks
Sugar	1 tablespoon
Syrup	1 tablespoon

Cakes, candy, chocolate, cookies, pies, etc. contain excessive calories and cannot be readily reduced to serving portions.

METHOD #2: ONE GLORIOUS MEAL A DAY

In working with overweight individuals, I have found that many of them give little thought to what and how much they eat. These individuals are never really hungry; but at the same time they are never quite satisfied. They normally eat out of force of habit, and often miss meals because "something came up" during their usual eating times. When this happens, their next meal is usually larger than it should be, and thus a certain balance is achieved in their daily intake of food.

Most of these individuals report that dinner is their most enjoyable meal. It doesn't seem to bother them that they may have missed one or both of the days earlier meals so long as dinner is large and satisfying. For these individuals I have found that scheduling one meal a day works wonders. Instead of gulping down a breakfast which they rarely want and eating lunch only because they have an hour to kill at midday, these individuals would rather eat a rich, substantial, and flavorful dinner.

If this one meal is properly balanced and sufficient quantities are eaten, one glorious meal a day will satisfy both physical and psychological needs. This method also works well if you know you are going out to dinner and probably will eat and drink more than you should. By skipping breakfast and lunch on those days, you will not have to restrict your dinner intake as you normally would.

If this method of maintaining weight sounds intriguing, by all means use it—either partially or wholly. You may find that one good meal is more satisfying and more easily controllable than three smaller meals.

Don't be put off by previous experiences. In the past you may have found that a few hours after missing a meal you felt weak and tired. This was due to a lowering of your blood sugar and probably was the result of improper diet. Now that you will be eating properly, and using one or more of the methods contained in this chapter, undesirable side effects will be minimal.

You may use the Daily Consumption Charts (A and B) found under Method #1 to help you in putting your meals together, or you may use the following Daily Meal Menu as a guide.

When using this method of weight maintenance, you will quickly find that it is almost impossible to overeat. Most times you will find it necessary to have one or more snacks during the day to meet your required intake of food. This, of course, is perfectly alright so long as you eat the proper quantities of the various foods.

METHOD #3: LIMITING A FOOD FACTOR FOR CONTINUED SLENDERNESS

Another method of maintaining lowered weight is to limit one of the basic food factors normally eaten. Since protein is an essential food factor and is necessary for the growth and repair of body tissue, it should not be restricted for extended periods of time. Carbohydrates and fats on the other hand, although necessary for good

SAMPLE DAILY MENU
(One Meal Per Day)
—137 pound woman—

	Meat	Veg.	Fruit	Milk	Bread	Fat	Sugar
Cocktail: Bloody Mary			2				1
Snacks Before Meal: Nuts Celery, Raw Carrot, Pickles, etc.	0.5	0.5					
Hors'd Oeuvre: Pate de Foie on Toasted Triangles	0.5				2	0.5	
Appetizer: Shrimp Scampi	2	1				0.5	
Soup: French Onion Soup Gratinee		1		0.5	1	0.5	
Salad: Lettuce, tomato, radish, onion with Roquefort Dressing	0.5	0.5				0.5	
Wine: Ss. Emillion							1
Entree: Large Cut Roast Prime Rib	2						
Vegetables: Large Baked Potato with Butter 1 cup Green Peas with Onions 1 cup French Fried Squash		2 2			2 1	0.5 0.5	
Cheese/Fruit/Crackers	0.5		2		1		
Ice Cream, small serving				1			
Coffee or Tea with Milk & Sugar							1
TOTALS	6.0	7.0	4.0	2.0	7.0	3.0	3.0

health, can be restricted to varying degrees without any untoward effects.

Some people find that limiting the intake of one of these factors is more easily accomplished than any of the other methods. If you find this method appeals to you, decide which factor you can most easily limit. You need only limit one or the other factor (carbohydrates or fats) to maintain your lowered weight.

MAINTAINING YOUR WEIGHT WITH FEWER CARBOHYDRATES

Carbohydrates are found in many foods and can be quite easily restricted. You should limit carbohydrate intake in accordance with the following instructions to produce the best results. Formulate menus which satisfy you by using the Daily Food Charts (A and B, Method #1) as a basis. The following Carbohydrate Content Chart indicates the number of grams of carbohydrate contained in one serving of each of the different food categories.

CHART C: CARBOHYDRATE CONTENT

	Number of grams of carbohydrate found in one serving of the following:
Meat	0
Vegetable	7
Fruit	10
Milk	12
Bread	15
Fat	0
Sugar	Contains excessive carbohydrates and must be completely elimated from daily food intake.

To determine your daily intake of food proceed as follows:

Restricted Carbohydrates

For men: pick the weight you wish to maintain. Multiply this weight by 1.1. This will give you the total number of grams of carbohydrate which may be eaten in any one 24-hour period. By referring to the Carbohydrate Content Chart, you will be able to determine how many servings of the various category foods you are permitted to eat so as not to exceed the permitted number of grams daily.

For Women: proceed as for men but multiply your maintenance weight by .88 to determine the total grams of carbohydrate permitted daily.

Note: Both men and women may eat as much food as desired during any one particular day so long as the total number of grams of carbohydrate does not exceed the recommended level.

REDUCING FATS TO STAY SLIM

Fat intake is often more difficult to control than is carbohydrate intake. Many foods are a combination of fat and protein, while others are prepared with fat (i.e., butter, oil, etc.) This many times results in you eating fats without even knowing it. You must therefore restrict certain fat-containing foods from your diet, while limiting others. The following Fat Content Chart indicates the number of grams of fat contained in one serving of each of the different food categories:

CHART D: FAT CONTENT

	Number of Grams of fat found in one serving of the following:
Meat	5
Vegetable	0
Fruit	0
Milk	10
Bread	10
Fat	5
Sugar	0

RESTRICTED FATS

To determine your daily intake of food follow the same steps as for the carbohydrate restricted method. However, for men, multiply maintenance weight by .56 and for women by .44 to determine the exact number of grams of fat permitted each day.

In the fat-restricted, as in the carbohydrate-restricted method, you may eat as much food as you desire so long as you do not exceed the number of grams of fat permitted daily.

HOW TO LOSE POUNDS BEFORE
THEY BECOME PERMANENT

During your post-program period there will undoubtedly be times when, for one reason or another, you fail to pay attention and find that you have eaten improperly. When this occurs, don't be discouraged. By utilizing either of the following procedures you will be able to reverse any undesirable effects and eliminate the possibility of regaining weight quickly and easily.

HOW THE ENERGY EXPENDER OFFSETS
INACTIVITY OR OVERINDULGENCE

Maintaining one's weight is not much different from losing weight. A balance must exist between energy expenditure and energy intake in the form of calories. Now that you are slender, you will undoubtedly be more energetic and therefore perform more physical activities than before. When this is the case, there is no need for prescribed exercise or for increasing energy expenditure through additional expenders. On the other hand, if for some reason your physical activities are restricted because of disability, work routine, inclement weather, etc., or your food intake is greater than it should be, you should immediately increase your energy expenders proportionately. This is essential if you are to maintain your lowered weight. Don't put it off! If you find your physical activities are being lessened, immediately add a new energy expender to your routine. On a temporary basis, one new expender used for one week will more than offset a full day of inactivity or one day's dietary indiscretions. By continuing indefinitely with the expender you will find that isolated restrictions in activity do little harm, and that occasional excesses in dietary intake are of little consequence. If however, you find yourself in doubt as to whether or not you are being active enough or eating properly, add another expender. It will preclude your gaining weight in the future.

HOW TO USE THE MEGATETIC TABLET TO MAINTAIN YOUR WEIGHT

In a previous chapter I stated that prolonged use of any medication, without a doctor's prescription, was unwise and potentially detrimental. I herewith restate that caution, but also must advise you that occasional, intermittent use of the Megatetic tablet by normal, healthy individuals will not cause any problems and will produce desired results.

If you faithfully follow the recommendations found in the preceding sections of this chapter you will find no reason to rely on the Megatetic tablet or on additional energy expenders. If, on the other hand, you find that you have been indiscreet and circumstances make it difficult for you to further restrict your intake of food or increase your physical activities, you should then turn to the Megatetic tablet. Follow the directions contained in Chapter 5 for its proper use, and you will not have to worry about regaining those unwanted pounds.

HOW PETER G. HELPED REVERSE THE EFFECTS OF OVEREATING

Peter G. is a young account executive and due to the nature of his position he finds himself frequenting numerous restaurants for the purpose of entertaining clients.

Because of this, Peter originally chose Method #2 for his post-program procedure and found it to work best for him, Unfortunately, on several occassions Peter found himself entertaining two different clients on the same day. In order to preclude offending either client Peter found himself eating more than he should. To prevent his regaining weight (he had originally lost 42 pounds) Peter used the Megatetic tablet at both meals and therefore reversed any of the effects which may have resulted from his overindulgence.

Today, Peter tells me that on occasion he has found it useful to rely on the Megatetic tablet, especially when circumstances force him to eat more than his post-program procedure permits.

WHY ROGER A. CHOSE ONE MEAL A DAY

When Roger first sought help for his overweight problem he was 48 years old, weighed 287 pounds, and was 5' 11" tall. Roger was married, and had two grown children both of whom had families of their own. For a 48-year-old man Roger had achieved a modicum of success. He had started out as a salesman for a large department store chain and had gradually but steadily improved his position until at the time he first entered the Center he had become manager of the Palm Beach store.

On a normal business day Roger did not eat breakfast, but did eat both lunch and dinner. The top floor of his store was a French restaurant which served as a meeting place for many of the store's customers. Roger normally would have his lunch in this restaurant since it was so convenient. He enjoyed the rich food immensely and often, when required to work later than usual, would find himself having dinner in this same restaurant.

Although his normal routine allowed Roger to take dinner with his wife, the meals she prepared were no less fattening than those of the restaurant. Mrs. A. had come to know Roger's craving for rich and varied foods. Since her children no longer occupied her time she had become an excellent gourmet cook. She often spent several hours preparing a meal for her husband—knowing how much he would enjoy it. Unfortunately Mrs. A. usually made more than adequate amounts, and Roger (not wanting to hurt his wife's feelings) would dutifully consume more than he actually needed. His wife, on the other hand, had little desire to eat because she had continually tasted the food as she was preparing it. This, in conjunction with the overly large portions and frequent restaurant meals were putting more and more weight on Roger's heart.

Although Roger's position afforded him ample time to partake in sports and other physical activities, the mental and emotional drain on his energies usually left Roger in a depleted state. His position required him to attend more social events than he really cared to, but he knew the importance of making an appearance at these often charitable affairs. Over the years, as Roger's weight steadily increased, his ability to fight it . . . to attempt to lose weight, decreased.

Except for a rather insignificant and accidental occurrence, Roger probably never would have sought assistance with his weight problem. It was during one of Florida's many storms, more violent than usual, that the electric power at the department store failed. Although the emergency lighting went on, the escalators and elevators weren't working. Roger, who was just arriving at the store at the time of the power failure, was forced to walk up to his offices on the third floor. By the time he arrived at his destination, he knew he had to do something about his weight. He could feel the tightness around his chest, the inability to catch his breath and the pounding of the blood vessels in his ears. Roger thought he would have a coronary at any moment. It was because of this fear that Roger made up his mind to get into shape.

After our usual pre-program examinations, Roger was put on two succeeding 30-day programs. For Roger the first days of the program were easy. He felt no great desire for food. Only during the third week did he find himself hard put to stay with it. But stay with it he did! By the end of his second 30-day program Roger had reduced his weight to 198; a total loss of 89 pounds.

The change in his appearance was dramatic; Roger decided he was happy at that weight and that he did not wish to lose any more. He had followed the Megatetic program completely and was more than satisfied with the results. When questioned about the post-program procedure Roger told me that he would follow the One Meal a Day method of weight maintenance. He explained that he still had a great desire for "good" food. He felt that breakfast and lunch weren't essential to him, but he truly loved a varied and appealing dinner. Since most of the social functions he attended, and the entertaining he and his wife did were in the evening, Roger felt that enjoying dinner was more important than eating three restricted meals a day.

Mrs. A. still enjoys gourmet cooking (although she has learned to prepare smaller servings) and Roger routinely walks up to his third-floor office as part of his daily Energy Expender. He feels younger and healthier than he has in many years and he now has the energy to participate in several physical activities that he had neglected since he was a young man. I don't think Roger will ever again allow himself to become overweight.

12 | HOW TO ENJOY EVERY DAY

Since you are an individual with unique needs and desires, it would be both foolhardy and presumptuous of me to offer specific ways to enjoy yourself. At the same time, however, there are several generalizations which can be made. Hopefully, your interpretation and utilization of these generalizations will assist you in maintaining a positive and enjoyable outlook.

LIKING YOURSELF IS ALL IMPORTANT

During the time you were overweight, there were, most likely, several activities or events which you didn't particularly enjoy.

Many previously overweight patients have reported that they felt uncomfortable and self-conscious whenever circumstances required them to wear clothes which did not, at least partially, conceal their obesity (i.e., swimming, tennis, etc.). Other patients have stated that besides the unflattering clothes, the physical activities in themselves were points of embarassment. They felt clumsy and awkward because of their excess weight. Although many continued to be involved in physical activities, they felt that they were missing much enjoyment because of these feelings.

If you will think about these statements for a moment, you will quickly realize that it wasn't the clothing or the activity which was embarassing, but rather the way in which these patients saw themselves. In truth, they were unhappy with their own physical appearance and therefore didn't wish to expose themselves to others, for fear of ridicule.

Today however, you are slender and deserve to be proud of your accomplishment. No longer should you restrict your activities, or the types of clothing you wear. Consciously . . . like yourself, and you will find it easy to like your surroundings. Each and every day you will find enjoyment in new activities and relationships; but first like yourself.

BEING TOO SERIOUS CAN OFTEN HINDER ENJOYMENT

Although "paying attention to business" is an essential ingredient for success in almost any endeavor; it can sometimes be overdone. Now that you have achieved your goal, I am sure that you never want to be fat again. However, you should not be too hard on yourself. By all means, "pay attention to business"; but don't overdo it. Being too serious can hinder your enjoyment.

The Megatetic Post-Program Procedure has been designed to permit great flexibility. In this way it can be adapted to your particular needs. From time to time you may find that you've exceeded the limits; have overindulged. By all means, get back on the track, but don't be too strict, and don't become depressed. Enjoy your dietary program by not becoming too serious; and you will be able to live with it forever.

ENJOYING THOSE PARTIES

Getting together with friends is always enjoyable, but much of the pleasure will be lost if you have to continually limit your food and drink. One way to prevent social gatherings from becoming prolonged torture is by being prepared.

It only takes a few minutes to analyze the kind of party you will be attending. Consider what food and drink will be served and then decide how much you will eat or drink. If you feel that you may overdo it at the party, you would be smart to restrict yourself to only one meal that day. Do not eat during the day so that you can enjoy the food and drink which will be served at the party.

If somehow, even with these precautions you eat or drink too much . . . don't be overly concerned. The next day initiate a new energy expender and within a few days your overindulgence will be nullified. In this way, by being prepared, you will be able to enjoy those social gatherings without putting on pounds.

HOW TO EAT OUT AND STILL STAY SLENDER

Going out to restaurants is perhaps one of the most enjoyable pastimes. Trying new foods and experiencing exotic flavors can definitely provide great pleasure. You should have no problem dining out if you will only follow the recommended food intake for your weight and sex.

When handed a menu, take your time to study it before ordering. Analyze the different foods offered in terms of the various food categories. Break down particular items into their component parts and then decide which foods best fulfill your requirements.

By using a little restraint you will be able to enjoy eating out without gaining a pound.

JANICE T.: A POSTSCRIPT

One of the very first patients ever put on the Megatetic Program was Janice T. She was 25 years old, 5′ 4½″ and weighed 154 lbs. At the time, Janice was single. She worked as a legal secretary for one of the larger law firms in the area, and was apparently quite competent as she once remarked that she was the highest paid secretary in the firm. Unfortunately, Janice was required to work in one of the private offices, and rarely came in contact with clients or visitors. Because of this, Janice paid little attention to her appearance. At one point, another secretary, whom Janice felt was not as qualified as she was, was given a promotion. Since the new position afforded several benefits, Janice was considerably disturbed at having been passed over. It was at that point that Janice decided to do something about her obesity and her appearance. She was very conscientious and in less than a month had achieved her weight-loss goal. In addition, Janice began to take an interest in clothes and cosmetics; she even took an adult education course in fashion design.

In a few months the change in Janice's appearance was so great as to be unbelievable. In a short time she was no longer required to make office visits and was therefore discharged. A few months ago Janice unexpectedly dropped in at the office. She related the following story:

"After losing all that weight I began to feel good about myself. I wanted to meet people and go out on dates. Unfortunately my employers didn't seem too interested in my changing positions. I therefore found another job with a different firm. The work was about the same, but I came in contact with lots of new people. I began to date one of the junior partners and last month he proposed to me. We're going to be married next month and I want to invite you to the wedding. Without you and your diet program I'd probably still be working in that back room."

INDEX